Praise for *Break Through with Breathwork*

"Jim Morningstar has written a heartfelt masterwork of breath-centered therapeutic support. He draws on an expansive knowledge of multicultural breath practices throughout history and many years of his own deep personal work and professional practice. The result is a valuable contribution at the growing edge of modern therapy, and a revolutionary blueprint combining mind/body healing and the latest findings in brain research."

> —Tav Sparks, author of *The Power Within: Becoming, Being, and the Holotropic Paradigm* and director of Grof Transpersonal Training

"Jim Morningstar is a wise and visionary healer, who knows the ways of the body and the heart. His work opens from trauma to well-being, from past to radiant present."

> —Jack Kornfield, Buddhist teacher and author of *The Roots of Buddhist Psychology*

"A profound and comprehensive book based on extensive experience as therapist and trainer, including new scientific research and informative models from biology and sociology, thus underlining the central role of conscious breathing in daily life and healing work. A must-read for therapists in any area of personal development and healthcare."

> —Dr. Wilfried Ehrmann, international trainer in integrative breathwork and author of *Manual of Breath Therapy* and *Coherent Breathing: Aligning Breath and Heart*

"Dr. Jim Morningstar is one of the real pioneers in breathwork. In his new book he offers a good illustration of how Therapeutic Breathwork represents a new form of interactive healing that benefits both client and therapist. With its comprehensive theory and overview of breathwork, it is an essential contribution to breathwork as a whole."

> —Gunnel Minett, psychologist and author of *Exhale: An Overview of Breathwork* and *How to Grow a Healthy Mind*

"A pioneer in breathwork and energetics, Jim Morningstar inspires the respect and admiration of practitioners in the field. His work with integrative techniques and his insights have encouraged my personal and professional growth."

—Dr. Belisa Vranich, clinical psychologist,
media personality, and author of *Breathe*

"Throughout *Break Through with Breathwork*, Jim Morningstar presents actual case studies that add a wonderful human touch, as well as an explanation based on neuroscience for the changes that he has seen in clients during his experience as a breathwork practitioner. This book is one of the few of its kind that demonstrates the safe and effective usage of faster than normal breathing in professional practice. *Break Through with Breathwork* should be read by anyone interested in evolving modern counseling techniques to keep pace with the growing need to help people face the challenges of life today. Both professionals and nonprofessionals alike will be struck by Jim Morningstar's clarity, involvement, and attention to detail, which is such an integral part of healing. A must-read! I highly recommend it."

—Shirley Telles, MBBS, MPhil, PhD (neurophysiology), DSc (yoga),
director of Patanjali Research Foundation in Haridwar, India

"Jim Morningstar was one of the first therapists in America to understand and explore the connection between mind, body, breath, and emotions. His approach, called Therapeutic Breathwork, has proven to be extremely effective in the field of trauma recovery, especially in cases where prescription medications and talk therapy have failed. His model of the six major breathing patterns and their link to basic body themes is truly unique and nothing short of brilliant. This chapter alone makes his newest book *Break Through with Breathwork* a must-read for every breathworker and all healthcare practitioners. And it offers invaluable support and genuine inspiration to all of us on the path of personal growth and spiritual development."

—Dan Brulé, author of *Just Breathe: Master Breathwork
for Success in Life, Love, Business and Beyond*

"In the coming years we are going to see a greater focus on the use of breathing to bring about healing in counseling and clinical mental health practice. Jim's extensive personal and professional experience of breathwork places him in an ideal position to introduce breathwork to those new to these practices. And for the more experienced practitioner this book provides plenty of stimuli for further personal integration and professional growth."

—Lloyd Lalande, PhD, clinical breathwork researcher and trainer and lecturer in clinical mental health counseling

"Jim Morningstar walks the talk and breathes the breath. He is a leading figure in breathwork today. If you aspire to use breathwork in counseling, this breakthrough book is your resource."

—Dr. Joy Manné, author of *Soul Therapy and Family Constellations*

"Jim has created a wonderful guide to help empower practitioners from all walks to add breathwork to their toolbox. This type of breathing breaks through old, no longer useful patterns while helping the practitioner and client create a healthy new vibrant way of life. Jim instills the confidence and knowledge to begin this great life adventure of breathwork personally and professionally."

—Lauren Cafritz, breath facilitator, lecturer, and teacher

BREAK THROUGH
with BREATHWORK

Jump-Starting Personal Growth
in Counseling and the Healing Arts

Jim Morningstar, PhD

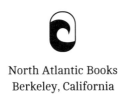

North Atlantic Books
Berkeley, California

Published by   Cover photo © iStockphoto.com/isurasaki
North Atlantic Books   Cover design by Nicole Hayward
Berkeley, California   Book design by Happenstance Type-O-Rama

Printed in the United States of America

Break Through with Breathwork: Jump-Starting Personal Growth in Counseling and the Healing Arts is sponsored and published by the Society for the Study of Native Arts and Sciences (dba North Atlantic Books), an educational nonprofit based in Berkeley, California, that collaborates with partners to develop cross-cultural perspectives, nurture holistic views of art, science, the humanities, and healing, and seed personal and global transformation by publishing work on the relationship of body, spirit, and nature.

Photographs in Chapter Five were originally published in *Spiritual Psychology* (1980), Transformations Incorporated; copyright Jim Morningstar. Reprinted with permission.
Illustrations in Chapter Three by Clare W. Graves; previously published in *Spiritual Psychology* (1980), Transformations Incorporated; copyright Jim Morningstar. Reprinted with permission.
Illustrations in Chapter Five by Emma Cofod.

MEDICAL DISCLAIMER: The following information is intended for general information purposes only. Individuals should always see their health-care provider before administering any suggestions made in this book. Any application of the material set forth in the following pages is at the reader's discretion and is his or her sole responsibility.

North Atlantic Books' publications are available through most bookstores. For further information, visit our website at www.northatlanticbooks.com or call 800-733-3000.

Library of Congress Cataloguing-in-Publication data
is available from the publisher upon request.

1 2 3 4 5 6 7 8 9 Sheridan 22 21 20 19 18 17

Printed on recycled paper

North Atlantic Books is committed to the protection of our environment. We partner with FSC-certified printers using soy-based inks and print on recycled paper whenever possible.

Acknowledgments

This book is for those in the healing arts who have felt a calling to discover and live their greater vision, who know there is more than can be learned in books, and who require essential connection with others. It is dedicated to those who sense their vocation to work with people is more than reinforcing their normality, but embraces championing their uniqueness. It is for those who have tasted the satisfaction of inspiring others to honor their larger mission in life and have felt great pride in seeing them reach for their true potential in spite of setbacks and challenges. It is gifted to those who have glimpsed the truth of the mirror that their clients hold up to them and are humbled by the teaching they receive in the process. It is these individuals who know their passion to serve others is also their path of self-awareness and inner discovery, who have experienced being energized by their service and seek to have that be their daily and lifelong experience. It is to these courageous souls whom I dedicate this book as a road map to understanding the history, dynamics, tools, and challenges that their profession provides. I honor those who are willing to risk getting beyond institutionalized roles and embrace their true being as they are helping others do the same. I also dedicate this book to the Spirit of Breath, which has informed, sustained, and transported me each day to be fully present in my body and my relationships while staying tuned to the transmissions of guidance that speak to my heart. It is this spirit that teaches all who are open to follow the rainbow bridge of breath to all levels of their being and dimensions of their soul; the breath connects us from top to bottom, Father Sky to Mother Earth united in the sacred heart of the Human.

Finally, I acknowledge those pioneers in the healing arts who have helped usher in a new era of whole-person transformation, who have broken from tradition to help forge new pathways into our cocreated future, who have passed on discoveries they have made by putting themselves through the trial by fire, and who have not only walked their talk but ushered others on their paths. Some of these are teachers of mine, including Clare W. Graves, Alexander Lowen, Cheng Man Chang, Leonard Orr, and my wife, Joan Morningstar. I am also grateful beyond measure for the guides and Guidance that have been with me every step on my path.

Jim Morningstar, PhD

Contents

Foreword

On a lovely summer morning in 2004, amidst the beautiful countryside of Estonia, I first watched Jim Morningstar facilitating a breathwork session. Estonia is a magical country that regained its independence without any bloodshed from the then Soviet Union in the late evening of August 20, 1991, through the unprecedented "Singing Revolution" that took place over four years. Imagine that courage, that innovation, and also the pain of fifty-one years of oppression—three from Nazi Germany and forty-eight from the Soviet Union. The people in Estonia both were amazingly vital and contained lingering trauma, and the people with whom we were working were craving healing and growth. The atmosphere was imbued with intensity, vibrant life force, repressed emotion, unshackled feelings, and unchartered territory. I was in awe of each Estonian.

Jim was working with a man who was obviously bound up by years of grief, confusion, rage, and repression, while feeling electricity and excitement for new pathways of living. I watched for five minutes and became an immediate fan of Jim's work. I witnessed a combination of nuanced attunement, tenderness, empowering support, deep wisdom, strength, and faith in this man's capacity and value. I saw Jim guiding him through rage, pain, the need of a body/heart/mind/spirit that wanted to open to the full potency of his life force, sexuality, relational capacity, power, creativity, and gifts. The process was sublime, manifold, creative, and harmonious. It was a coherent integration of all this man was bringing to this powerful moment of longing for expression, wholeness, and actualization.

It would not be an overstatement to say that the beautiful Estonian who was in Jim's capable hands worked through months and years of inner experiences in one breathwork session.

We all begin and end life with a breath. Everything that we experience, give, receive, grow, develop in ourselves, and love begins with each of us taking that first breath when we are born. It is then maintained and nourished by each breath through every moment of our lives. The implications of that are far more complex and multidimensional than we have integrated into mainstream life and popular culture. The biological, medical, emotional, cognitive, neural, philosophical, humanistic, and spiritual implications of this, while articulated and practiced for millennia, are just now in the late twentieth and early twenty-first century being explored and validated by science. What is powerful to consider, and what there is now ample validating research for, is that the quality of each breath is the single most powerful thing we can do to cultivate our physical, emotional, cognitive, and spiritual well-being.

Certainly it was the breath itself, it was the willing Estonian consciously partnering the breath that created the powerful transformation that I witnessed that day and that I have seen variations of in thousands of sessions facilitated by me, Jim, and courageous committed breathworkers all over the globe. And certainly Jim has created this book in service of the breath and its potential impact for individuals and even humanity at large. Yet I think to understand the magnitude of what you are about to read, I need to say a little more about Jim, and maybe more importantly about his example, so that you can understand the anatomy, potency, and skill of a person who befriends and partners the breath for a long time and has the intelligence, love, and courage to bring breathwork into therapeutic and healing spaces.

Watching Jim Morningstar facilitate any breathwork session is always a deeply touching, inspiring, educational experience, and it usually turns out to be personally transformative for me.

In every session he embodies vision, skill, and care.

...vision, not only about how someone can move through whatever difficulties and openings they need to but also the faithful vision that their life has undeniable purpose that can be contacted and lived from.

...*skill* that is not only derived from disciplined practice of intelligent methodologies but also such refinement that, like the virtuosity of a world-class violinist, it spans an expansive continuum of breadth and depth that can support emergent forms of creativity and wisdom.

...*care* that is not only the unconditional positive regard that Carl Rogers taught us about but also an attunement so sensitive it nourishes and waters the most wounded, withered, and terrified parts of ourselves into health and life.

These are the feelings, images, and awarenesses that arise whenever I think of Jim. And now he has managed to transmit that same level of vision, care, and skill into a courageous and comprehensive book that articulates and opens a doorway that humanity longs for and needs—to contact the depth of what we are, to live from that depth, and to have that depth reflected in all the actions of our daily lives. There is a vision here: first, that every individual that breathes consciously can have a life of deep meaning, purpose, and fulfillment and, second, that humanity can open to a greater compassion and understanding of one another and experience a visceral fundamental respect and honoring of the uniqueness of each person and their connectedness with one another.

He has written a book with such transparency, clarity, simplicity, and accessibility. How is it possible? If you want to know what developing a lifelong relationship with conscious breathing can look like in an ordinary human life, and in a daily way, I can't urge you enough to read every word of this precious and groundbreaking book.

In his acknowledgments Jim recognizes his teachers and says of them, "Finally, I acknowledge those pioneers in the healing arts who have helped usher in a new era of whole-person transformation, who have broken from tradition to help forge new pathways into our cocreated future, who have passed on discoveries they have made by putting themselves through the trial by fire, and who have not only walked their talk but ushered others on their paths." Well, choosing to take a lifelong journey with conscious breathing has made Jim one of those people.

That this foreword may appear to be more about Jim than the actual power of breath is a testimony to the field of breathwork. Breathwork practitioners can't help but love their clients unconditionally and see them as beautiful, noble, and richly endowed with all kinds of possibilities. And if we are committed to that in others, we are humbled into living an examined life that transforms our relationship with ourselves and others from unconscious fear-based living to conscious love-based living, one breath at a time. Over time, it will bring forth for examination all parts of us that hold ourselves back from fully expressing our gifts and potency. It will reveal ways that we harm ourselves and others or create unnecessary separation and suffering. It points out to us ways that we are in competition with others and ways that we turn away from giving and receiving love … and so much more.

Breathwork readily opens loving, powerful, ethical, wise doorways to a healthy, expanded, and integrated soma, psyche, and soul. This is what Jim has modeled for us. This is what breath is inviting all breathworkers to do. This is what healing practitioners can learn. This is what all of us can learn to take into any vocation, including parenting, friendships, sexual relationships, and spiritual vocations. It takes patience, courage, dedication, willingness to be changed, attention, study, practice, intention, strength, and love.

It is so worth it. We are talking about the fundamental basis and nutrient of life … what we are and what we can become.

I take a breath with you now and each moment.

With love and blessings,

JESSICA DIBB
Global Professional Breathwork Alliance, codirector
Unified Global Breathwork Field, founder
Inspiration Community and Consciousness School, founder and director

April 16, 2017 (Easter Sunday, the Seventh Night of Passover)

Introduction

The more you believe in the power of thought, and the more you listen to your breath, the greater changes you can create in your life.

—STIG ÅVALL SEVERINSEN, *Breatheology*

It may seem to be stating the obvious to note that all counselors and their clients breathe during their sessions together. Yet it's important to bring attention to this simple truth because until now the quality of how we breathe has largely been ignored in the healing process, or at best seen as a sideline to improved functioning of the client. Adjuncts to counseling that focus on healthy breathing have been recommended in some cases to clients to improve general mood and energy levels, and healthy breathing practices, such as yoga and *T'ai Chi*, are becoming more popular. But even these are relatively rare as a general component of counseling or other healing modalities and take place outside the consulting room. A longstanding demarcation between healing the mind and emotions versus care for the body has separated counseling from physical health domains. I believe this is to the detriment of both fields, but more poignantly to the detriment of clients. This for me is more than an interesting hypothesis. It has been borne out in my life work as a therapist since 1972.

After years of doctoral training and a National Institute of Mental Health (NIMH) clinical internship as a psychotherapist, I was despairing at the thought of continuing at the snail's pace of most verbal therapeutic processes that focused on mental changes and only haphazardly produced lasting behavioral changes in clients' lives. It was not until I was introduced to body-oriented therapies in the early seventies that the lightbulb went on. I saw how I and my clients in turn could embody changes in our lives that were palpable and lasting in much shorter periods of time than resulted from just talking about our issues.

The Importance of Breath and Good Breathing Habits

To breathe is to live. *How* we breathe has a most profound influence on the quality of our life. Breathing correctly is the key to living fully. Most Westerners suffer from chronic improper breathing habits that are not immediately obvious. We breathe about seven million breaths a year, and the long-term effects of poor breathing are cumulative. They reduce not only the quality of vitality in our daily experience but can lead to a weakening of our entire system and serious health issues. We can take health for granted until we encounter serious problems. It has been estimated that 60 percent of all emergency transports in larger American cities involve hyperventilation or other breath-related disorders.[1] Research suggests that ten to twenty-five percent of the U.S. population suffers from breath-related illness every year. Improper breathing weakens and disharmonizes almost every major system in our bodies and makes us more susceptible to chronic and acute diseases of all kinds: infections, constipation, respiratory illness, digestive problems, ulcers, depression, sexual disorders, sleep disorders, fatigue, headaches, poor blood circulation, and premature aging. Many researchers believe bad breathing contributes to cancer and heart disease. Proper breathing can keep the systems of the body functioning in harmony, signal us about imbalances in our energy and help us correct them, and thereby be a perfect companion on route to our health and happiness.

Though in all cultures throughout history breath has been held as the most important factor in physical health as well as emotional stability and spiritual development, it receives little or no attention in our educational system, including medical training.[2] Proper breath training requires qualities in which modern Westerners are underdeveloped: focused attention, relaxation, internal awareness, and perseverance. Even healthy people often breathe only about a third of the oxygen they need to function optimally. The air we breathe is about five times larger by volume than that of the food we ingest and the liquid we drink. On the other side, seventy percent of the body's waste products are eliminated through the lungs and thirty percent through urine, feces, and skin.

We Can Change How We Breathe

We can change the quantity and quality of how we breathe. Dennis Lewis[3] cites that people have been trained in six to twelve months to increase the range of their diaphragms two to three times their capacities. But it is not just the amount of air we breathe that affects us. It is the balance in our breathing that determines whether our breath is giving us the correct proportions of oxygen and carbon dioxide to maximize the nurturance of our bodies. Researcher Peter Litchfield[4] notes that breathing regulates the pH balance of our body. I was amazed when I worked with Peter that within a few deregulated breaths the oxygen/carbon dioxide balance of my breathing was altered. He notes that deregulated breathing has a dramatic and profound effect on health and performance. In fact, most Americans do a type of "over-breathing" because of chronic tension in their breathing mechanism and attitudes in their minds. They develop a wrong combination of breathing rate and depth. The cure is not as simple as "relaxation" or "breathing more." Coming back to harmony with one's body and listening to find the right breath for the right activity is an eminently learnable skill. First we must recognize there is something to correct and then have the willingness to do something about it.

What Makes Breathwork a Unique Contribution to the Healing Arts?

Breathwork is the science and art of breath awareness and breath modulation. It is directed toward releasing dysfunctional patterns of physical, emotional, and mental functioning and bringing greater harmonious integration of one's network of life systems from the neurological to the spiritual—literally to feel more comfortable in one's skin. Therapeutic Breathwork™ has brought together time-honored healing traditions with contemporary breakthroughs in mind-body therapies.

Sitting in a room together in any therapeutic setting, the helper and client are each inhaling and exhaling one million particles with every breath and sharing their cocreated atmosphere on a molecular level. They are also transmitting radiant frequencies from their heart and brain centers that overlap and interact on an energetic level. Nonverbally they are communicating a myriad of signals through body posture and movement that they instinctively interpret and react to; verbally they convey information about their history, behaviors, beliefs, expectations, and aspirations that influence one another. Their contractual arrangement is for the therapist to assist the client in increasing his or her life functionality and satisfaction.

With all these levels of interaction, what does the therapist focus on, and how does the therapist intervene in the most useful ways? I believe the breath holds an obvious and overlooked key that is literally right under our noses. In any helping interaction, a rapport has to be established for a useful contract to be established and results achieved. Breath awareness has been an instantaneous indication for me as to the level of safety and comfort a client has in their body and the environment they share with me. My breathing and body posture shifts with the meeting of any new person—this is something that happens with all of us. If I am conscious of my interaction, I can immediately begin putting myself and the other person at ease and establishing rapport. If I unconsciously mimic or amplify the fear they are signaling, putting myself or the client in a defensive posture, I have set up impediments to our rapport from the start. Awareness of my breathing as a caregiver is a key to my effectiveness in communicating with my client.

Usually within the first hour I am with clients, I ask them to report what they notice about their breathing. This takes some care in phrasing so that the client doesn't take my prompt as a criticism. I begin the teaching of breath awareness as a self-regulating biofeedback mechanism at the onset. This helps clients to become aware, not only with me but also in their lives, of when they start to constrict their breathing. They begin to see how this breath holding is most often associated with a fear reaction, conscious or unconscious. This awareness is then coupled with the skill of altering their breathing to produce more resourcefulness in any situation. This is usually as simple as breathing a bit more freely, oxygenating their muscle systems for action, taking their emotional system out of the fight/flight/freeze reactivity, and opening their minds to more resourceful responses rather than knee-jerk reactions. With breath awareness, clients become more adept at using verbal therapy because they notice when they begin to resist a topic or new insight. They take cues from me about accepting this awareness as a useful tool rather than more material about which to criticize themselves: "What's wrong with me? I'm not breathing properly!" Here is where the therapist's "unconditional positive regard" and skill, when combined with breath awareness, provides a more powerful tool for clients than either one alone.

This breath awareness becomes the foundation for the practices that I call *maintenance breathing skills*, which have been so influential for humans through millennia in bringing increased peace of mind and body. This is exemplified by *pranayama* in the yoga tradition and translated into contemporary parlance as mindfulness and coherent breathing. Coherent breathing entails slowing the breath to five to six breaths per minute for four minutes or more. The physiological effects are well documented by HeartMath research[5] for regulating the parasympathetic nervous system, lowering blood pressure (as approved by the FDA), and calming the mind. The therapist can play an instrumental role in introducing this to clients who would consider such practices as too esoteric or irrelevant to their lives to even attempt. It is the practical and immediately experienced effects of breath awareness that can open their minds to the benefits of additional regularly implemented practices. Increasing awareness of their own bodies can also prepare clients for more major lifestyle renovations, such as opening up to changes in their dietary and exercise habits.

Therapeutic Breathwork adds to the toolbox of breath awareness and maintenance breathing, by including and teaching the skills of sympathetic nervous system regulation. Through increasing the normal breathing rhythm in a safe, supportive setting for the purpose of harmonizing the emotional system, past traumas and emotional blockages can be relieved more directly than through years of "beating around the bush" in conventional therapy. The "bush" in this metaphor is an area of unconscious or "implicit-only" memory that has stored emotional reactivity through trauma that gets activated by environmental stimuli and produces feeling and behavioral responses unaligned with current circumstances (see Chapter Four). These are labeled by most untrained observers as overreactions. In extreme cases, these reactivated memories are experienced as flashbacks, which put individuals in another time and space that feel out of their control.

The elegance of Therapeutic Breathwork is that it helps reprogram traumatic responses by going directly to the limbic system where they are stored, rather than trying to enter by the doorway of the prefrontal cortex whose pathways to the experience have been blocked by the body's emergency control systems. When clients learn to use this type of breathing consciously, they regain the confidence in their own abilities to handle settings and circumstances that were previously paralyzing to them—situations as simple as having dinner with their family or as dynamic as performing before a large audience.

As reinforced by contemporary research, the human brain develops in relation to its environment and more specifically in dyadic interactions with significant others.[6] We are, at our core neurology, relational beings. To reprogram traumatic responses, there is no more powerful tool than dyadic interaction, which helps stabilize and calm a deregulated nervous system and restore a sense of safety in one's body. Therein lies the power of bringing breathwork into the healing relationship.

Throughout this book you will find personal accounts relevant to the content that were submitted by clients and practitioners; these stories relate their experiences with Therapeutic Breathwork sessions or reflect on the effects of Therapeutic Breathwork over time.

Personal Account

Jim D., an anesthesiologist, recounts in his words "how the transformational effect of breathwork in concert with focused psychotherapy took me on a nine-year journey from psychic fragmentation and severe cultural conditioning to personal wholeness and family and community-centeredness."

continues

"I explored spirituality, energy medicine, and martial arts prior to my engagement with focused and regular psychotherapy, and although these areas added 'tools' to my 'toolkit' of psychological stability, they did not offer the grounding, stabilizing, and integrative experiences that I encountered with breathwork when combined with the psychotherapy sessions. To ferret out the sources of personal internal tension and neurosis and examine them in the light of day is a natural process with psychotherapy. However, this sort of 'psychologic excavation' often results only in an intellectual understanding of these psychological tensions. Intellectual examination of emotional, often nonrational issues ultimately proves fruitless in that the intellectual examination does not trace these issues to their root in the autonomic nervous system of the patient (i.e., the fight-or-flight response). The use of conscious, connected breathing in the form of Therapeutic Breathwork allows the client and therapist to plumb the source of psychological tensions within the client's autonomic nervous system, essentially the spinal cord and brainstem. Conditioned, fearful responses to memories, thoughts, or situations represent 'reflex arcs' in the spinal cord and brain stem, which are expressed through the sympathetic nervous system. Breathwork trains the client to identify the feelings and deeply seated sources of neurosis and transform them holistically during the psychotherapy session. In my experience as a client as well as a practitioner of Therapeutic Breathwork, I can confidently testify that the psychological, emotional, and physical integration I sought in psychotherapy would not have been possible without the tools of breathwork."

Dyadic Breathwork: Something New Under the Sun

The first challenge for therapists in being an effective change agent and teacher of Therapeutic Breathwork skills is becoming safe and conversant with the nonlinear world of their own sympathetic nervous system. The interactive energetic systems in the consulting room require that therapists be clear enough of their own "emotional blind spots" to be effective guides for clients. The helper must have the courage to be helped to greater levels of vulnerability and sensitivity. The comfort zone of therapeutic distance must be set aside when doing our own work as a therapist. The goal is to increase awareness of our own unconscious or shadow parts to effect greater self-integration. It ranges from difficult to impossible to lead a client down this path when we have not trod it ourselves. The benefits many therapists have derived from accepting this challenge are a greater sense of personal vitality, increased ability to work with a variety of clients more deeply and effectively, and less compassion fatigue as a result.

I both serve and support my clients and see them also as mirrors in whom I witness the parts of me that are in process of healing. Through my practice of breathwork, I am well able to keep therapeutic boundaries (even more consciously) without distancing and labeling the client as sick or deviant. They energetically respond to collaborative work as opposed to being "worked on" as a specimen. I suspect most therapists would feel insulted by the insinuation that they think of, much less treat, their clients as "specimens." Nonetheless, when clients journeying into their areas of conflict and fear causes me as a therapist to subtly guard myself emotionally, often by retreating to mental interpretation, advice-giving, and/or protective body language (impeding my own breathing), I am conveying the subtle message of "You are sick, and I need to manage you." Many clients are all too willing to accept this label because they are not comfortable with their own feelings and have concluded something is wrong with them, as opposed to seeing their feelings as a form of emotional intelligence that is trying to communicate valuable messages. These signals can warn them before they engage in behaviors that get them less of what they really want. My job as a therapist is to help them free these messages from negative judgment and translate them into self-affirmation and productive action.

This challenge for me in my therapy training was monumental. I had learned to suppress almost all of my feelings as a child, causing me to be less than open to those who expressed them freely. I could understand intellectually the benefits of accepting one's feelings but was terrified to fully experience mine, mostly defaulting to family patterns of withdrawal or sarcasm. Only years of work in Gestalt and Bioenergetic sessions helped me incorporate increased safety with my feelings into my body. This was before breathwork started to become popular in the 1970s.

Breathwork added a new dimension to my self-awareness because of its direct access to the emotional body. Bioenergetics, the body-mind therapy I studied with Alexander Lowen, had already showed me how the experience of fear correlated with breath constriction. Breathwork's ability to go directly to emotional material while keeping the breath open and flowing left little recourse for my intellectual defenses.

During such periods of emotional upheaval and restructuring that accompany a change process, our lives can feel on the edge of "out of control." Indeed, the old methods of emotional control are loosened, and behaviors can appear impulsive or even dangerous to those who have an investment in keeping everything at status quo such as family members, friends, or coworkers. Having a helper and possibly a network of supporters who have gone through their own process of emotional recovery and who can provide stability and guidance is crucially important in staying on the road to growth, not veering into the ditch of hurtful behaviors or reactive regression. Therapeutic Breathwork combines the tools of breath awareness, slower than normal breathing (maintenance breathing), and faster than normal breathing, all masterfully designed to help with emotional and mental regulation *en route* to a life of greater freedom and satisfaction.

Personal Account

Ron, a veteran psychotherapist, used his personal healing with Therapeutic Breathwork to inspire him to become a certified professional breathworker and integrate breathwork into his therapy practice. He shared the following experience of deep healing of his lifelong vertigo issue at a breathworker training.

"Never before, in any form of therapy I had experienced, had I ever been able to break through a wall that appears when panic and dizziness occur. At this point, in whatever mode I might be working, something would halt

continues

the process (and my breathing, of course!), and I could not go any further. As I got deeper into this breathwork session, I encountered a deep sense of terror and blackness, and things began to spin. With encouragement I was able to keep aware of my breathing and stayed with the process despite my longing to bolt and a flurry of beliefs that only suffering, and no gain, awaited me in this encounter. In reviewing the journal entry I made after the session, I described what I was experiencing as being in a dark and terrifying hell. I was aware of recurring fears of suffocating that I have often felt with this kind of severe panic. I think I may have asked several times to be assured that I would not suffocate and die. I felt silly in asking but desperately needed to hear clear reassurance that I was not in any kind of life-threatening danger. I learned that I could be dizzy and afraid, even terrified, and that I could still breathe. As obvious a truth as I can see this is now, there was no level of consciousness that held this belief prior to this experience. My journal entry emphasized that this awareness was new on all levels.

"I remember feeling like I was sinking in some deep darkness and spinning out of control. I was deeply terrified that this would be some kind of never-ending purgatory that I was going to end up in where this suffering would never abate. On some level I believed that the only way to keep myself out of that endless suffering was to not let myself really enter this darkness. And here I was going deeper into the place that I worked so hard to avoid and actually could never penetrate in the past regardless of my intentions. As this sense of spinning through the darkness continued, I kept breathing and battling the fear and began to see some small glimmer of light that appeared to be off in the distance. I also felt like I could see a terrified younger version of myself that was just out of my reach for what seemed like a very long time. I seemed to be spinning down some dark tunnel, and then at one point I heard Michelle, my breathworker, say something like, 'We are having a rebirth over here.' I know that at some point Steve (the trainer) joined the process and encouraged me to breathe and come toward the light. This became more difficult in some way because as I got closer to the light the spinning seemed to intensify. When I finally

continues

came through into the light, I was still experiencing some strong dizziness and shakiness, but I was awed and comforted by the light. And to my surprise what I had been viewing as a terrified inner child in darkness now became a peacefully swaddled baby, and I had a profound sense of being supported in the light by what I felt were spirits around me. It also was significant for me that as I came through this birthing-type experience that Steve was there at the end and just tenderly held my face in his hands. That felt like one of the pieces that began to arrive for me to fill that painful empty void of loving male presence in my life.

"This process helped me deepen my peace with my deceased mother and take me a step forward in healing the wounds connected to my absent father. Somewhere along the way in this process I became aware that I had taken on my parents' fear of suffering. I believe that this was a way to try to have a connection with them, though with obvious limitations and consequences. I got clear that my parents were in their own lights and that I could love them eternally just as they are. This experience helped me tremendously and has deepened my understanding and ability in helping my clients in the ways they try to connect through 'shared symptoms' in a desperate effort to have a link in a large and sometimes scary world.

"The benefits for me in this session have been astounding. I realized that panic and vertigo had been like a wall that I could never penetrate. And through this one session alone I passed through that wall and began traveling the territory beyond. How incredible to be on the other side of something that I wondered if I could ever penetrate! This has provided hope and encouragement to me, especially at times when I get discouraged or doubtful if I will move through a particular issue, and I think that I have been better able to bring that kind of hopefulness to my clients, from an understanding and sincere place. At this point I did not believe that I would be able to bring breathwork to others, but it launched me along the way. To have a breakthrough like this creates so much excitement, hope, and curiosity to learn more and heal more that this has energized me forward in my own healing and in the ways that I assist others in their process."

Note to Professional Therapists and Practitioners in the Healing Arts

Therapeutic Breathwork is a complete tool kit of breathwork techniques for the clinician. We train to seek the right breath for the right healing and growth situations in one's practice. There is no one size fits all technique for every circumstance. As such we adapt traditional slower than normal breathing for centering, relaxation, and meditative purposes, natural breathing for the everyday flow of life, and faster than normal breathing for energy release and breakthrough work in trauma healing and personal growth. We have specialized in the faster than normal techniques about which there are far less written in the literature and research. Familiarity with these techniques is spreading, and we are in the forefront of adapting it and training its use for all the healing arts. Much of this book focuses on this astounding evolutionary work and the growing body of practice and research in its use.

Although 30-60 minute breathwork sessions are presented in formal and first-person accounts in the text, the faster than normal breathwork, as well as slower than normal breathing, is creatively adapted to standard clinical practice from one minute awareness processes to 20 minute release cycles. We do recommend that practitioners be trained in the 30-60 minute faster than normal breathing techniques to be conversant with this application when it is the exact tool needed to help release well entrenched holding patterns. Also this training sensitizes the practitioner to the subtleties of their own and their clients' breathing patterns in all circumstances. It has helped me and a vast variety of practitioners to be both sensitive and creative in using the power of breath in all healing work, even when it does not involve directly focusing on the breath. We invite you to experiment and explore with the techniques in this text for yourself and connect with appropriate training centers for support in their clinical usage.

Chapter 1

Breath in the Consulting Room

Breathing represents the movement of the Creative Life, which, in each moment, dissolves that which threatens to harden us, in order to give birth to a new form. Work on breathing represents a transformation of the whole man. One must understand that superficial breathing is an expression of the man who keeps himself from becoming a Person. The self blocks the path toward transcendence.

—KARLFRIED GRAF DÜRCKHEIM

Since the 1970s, there has been an explosion in the United States and other countries in the blending of ancient breathing techniques for health and awareness found in disciplines such as yoga and *T'ai Chi* with contemporary therapeutic practices, such as Dialectical Behavioral Therapy and mindfulness. The result has been the evolution of powerful and incisive healing and consciousness-changing modalities. This has given birth to the field of *breathwork*, which has promoted significant advances in medical and psychological domains (see research references in Appendix Three).

As one of the newly emerging tools of complementary medicine, breathwork has the daunting yet highly exciting task of blending the old and the new for the purpose of creating something better than either in isolation. There are many varied schools of using breath therapeutically. I am referring in this chapter to the schools that have emerged in the past quarter-century, which train practitioners to work directly with the breathing patterns of clients to help them more consciously achieve and sustain physical, emotional, mental, and spiritual well-being.

Breathwork reinforces a new paradigm in the field of professional counseling: whole-brain learning. It bridges both brain hemispheres and accesses brain stem, limbic system, and cerebral cortex functions. It thereby reaches deeper levels of human motivation and behavioral control. Incorporating breathwork into counseling takes us to the intersection of science and art. We can assist appropriate clients to learn *organically,* not just with their rational thinking. Issues of addiction, for example, require a profound shift in values and motivation that must be learned experientially, espoused organically (not just intellectually), and reinforced environmentally for healthy change to be enduring.[7]

We no longer live in world of Newtonian physics or black-and-white thinking, and nor do our clients. Treatment that accesses the dualities of male/female, right/left, intuitive/logical is not just interesting; at this point in time it is necessary to help restore wholeness to today's clientele.

Traditional and Contemporary Uses of Breathwork in Healing Arts

Breathing practices such as yoga and Taoist techniques have been used in Asia for centuries, not just for health maintenance but for diagnosis and cure. Off-shoots have been used in Western medicine for ease in childbirth (the Lamaze technique coaches mothers to use their breath in specific ways during the birthing process to facilitate the delivery and minimize discomfort), pain control (hypnosis has been used to help those with chronic pain follow their breath and reduce pain), and asthma relief (the Buteyko method[8] uses controlled breathing and breath holding to control the over-breathing and panic that can happen in an asthma attack).

Psychotherapeutic Application

More recently breathwork has been used to treat panic attacks, anxiety, and a variety of mental-health disorders and emotional trauma not reached by more cognitive therapies. Often medication—a primary treatment protocol of mental-health clinicians—does not relieve chronic tension; it only temporarily masks it. Breathwork is a tool that helps reach underlying limiting beliefs and habitual behaviors held in place by negative conditioning.

Practitioners may learn to teach both diaphragmatic belly-oriented and costal heart-centered techniques to access either the parasympathetic or the sympathetic nervous system for particular healing effects. Therapeutic Breathwork utilizes both slower than normal breathing and faster than normal breathing patterns as appropriate for clients' needs. The results of slower than normal breathing (four to five breaths per minute) have been well documented through the research of HeartMath, mindfulness, and yogic pranayama practices. I recommend and use these practices for daily maintenance and well-being. The benefits of faster than normal breathing (thirty to seventy breaths per minute) have been less researched and used clinically. This book is a guide to help those in the healing arts integrate such breathwork safely, successfully, and ethically into their work.

This kind of breathwork gives counselors the following, both personally and professionally:

- A technique for relieving stress

- A parameter for daily self-care level

- A doorway to spiritual awakening

- An adjunct to counseling to assist clients in relief from both acute and chronic emotional and psychological pain and in maintaining more balanced lifestyles

Personal Account

Clare is a psychotherapist whose personal experience with Therapeutic Breathwork led her to its use with her clients.

"What most intrigues me about breathwork is the experience of discovery and the natural healing that takes place in a breathwork session. I have witnessed and participated in discovery and healing in my twenty-plus years of practice as a traditional psychotherapist, but my experience of breathwork brings a whole new dimension to my understanding of healing. As an example, I have experienced sensations in my body related

continues

to anxiety and depression released in the process of my own breathwork sessions. After a session, I almost invariably feel a profound sense of peace, often without knowing the storyline attached to the healing. My conscious, connected breathing discovered the pain and was the vehicle of its release. Traditional psychotherapy is sometimes so attached to the storyline that the relief can be delayed in order to satisfy the intellectual understanding. I am grateful that I became introduced to breathwork for my own growth and to enrich my therapy practice for my clients."

Outline of a Breathwork Session

A first breathwork session typically involves ten to fifty minutes of clinical interview and issue definition. I include in this information gathering what clients know about the event of their birth as well as the emotional climate (i.e., the relationship between their parents as best they can surmise at the time of their birth). Frequently I get a brief description of their parents' histories also. Then after an introduction to the breathing technique and its relevance to their conditions and goals, we do approximately thirty minutes to an hour of concentrated connected breathing that works on the levels of body, mind, emotions, and spirit. Clients typically lie down flat on a mat or on cushions with a blanket nearby if needed during the session, but they can also be in a relaxed sitting position. The first part of the session involves briefly clarifying clients' intention, which may be fairly general (e.g., releasing tension in their bodies) or more specific (e.g., dealing with death of a family member). Clients may also state what kind of support they invoke for their work (e.g., "I'd like my maternal grandmother's blessing on my journey"). The breathworker then coaches them to connect their inhale with their exhale without pause in a faster than normal rhythm. The breathworker may demonstrate this, adjusting according to what will energize but not overwhelm the client. The breathworker allows the client to establish a rhythm and then instructs the client to continue breathing even when being coached by the breathworker. The breathworker coaches the client on maintaining a free and open rhythm. The middle portion of the session involves the client being coached to stay with the breath as physical, emotional, mental, or spiritual material surfaces. This may involve active movement and expression by the client. The point of the coaching is to increase the client's ultimate sense of safety, freedom, and aliveness. At times this involves a more dramatic release and at times a very peaceful "letting go." The final portion of the session is for integration of the material surfaced and grounding in the body. Affirmations and homework for the client may be given by the breathworker who assists the client in applying the results to the client's life and suggesting appropriate follow-up. Note that this is a generic outline of a session. I have never had two that are the same.

BODY

Learning how to sustain a relaxed yet full breathing rhythm through whatever tension arises in the body is a precious gift. Chronic holding patterns in muscle as well as connective tissue can be released without exterior manipulation. Once we learn this, we attain a lifelong method of tension relief. This is an art form and not a mechanical process. We must sense the right breathing pattern for the appropriate circumstances. Like any skill, it develops with practice.

MIND

Holding patterns in the body reflect continual messages of protection—fight/flight/freeze responses from the brain. If our beliefs are such that we see ourselves as unsafe in our bodies and our world, our bodies will respond accordingly. In counseling, we are looking for more than temporary relaxation states, but a more enduring sense of inner harmony, which leads to more resourcefulness in dealing with life challenges. Counseling ferrets out core beliefs, and more functional beliefs are paired with new states that the client is trained to access. We learn new tools for working with belief systems and practice anchoring them with physiological sensations. They are individually developed tools for the reconstruction of a new consciousness, which can include more affirmative self-talk and self-image, and they provide a daily reinforcement of a new level of enjoyment in life.

EMOTIONS

Every family teaches its members by example which forms of emotional expression are acceptable and which are not. These norms become so ingrained that changing their patterning is beyond the normal range of therapist and client skills, even though the effects may be restrictive or dysfunctional. Working directly with the emotion centers of the brain is outside most people's conscious awareness. Messages to these areas, however, can be altered and the healthy range of expression expanded. A breathwork session provides an arena for more than release; it links positive states with client-directed breathing.

SPIRIT

Breathwork's underlying philosophy is that the key to change is accepting active responsibility for our lives and having our spirit in the driver's seat, instead of being driven by past conditioning. This is not a process of speculation and philosophizing but rather of direct experience. Counselors do not dictate to clients their spiritual truths. Clients come to know their own spiritual truths directly by virtue of their courage to go past fears and self-doubts.

Cycle of Breath

A breathwork session often involves the following:

- A beginning in which one experiments and discovers how to sustain a connected full rhythm

- A middle period of building an energetic charge to a point of release

- An ending period during which the released energy is grounded and suggestions for application are integrated

Breath and Energy Releases

Holding patterns in the breath mechanism frequently date back to early life up to and including birth. Some people have somatic memories of their birth and the fear that generated their holding. But uncovering these memories is not necessary to the release process. There is a distinct difference in the ease and pleasure of the breath after the moment of breath release. This is most often followed by an energy release felt throughout the body. The physical sensations of this vary with individuals and relate to the dissolution of their chronic areas of suppression.

Breathwork Training for Counselors

Use of breathwork in counseling requires the skill and sensitivity of trained counselors who have gone through the process of learning the breathwork technique themselves. Breathwork can induce mild trance or nonordinary states of consciousness. With the direction of an adept therapist, clients can access material that might take them years to reveal—if ever—with traditional talk modalities. This requires the therapist to be conversant with such states, how to use the material (including memories, emotions, and physical sensations), and how to assist clients to integrate and sustain insight and behavioral change.

Stanislav Grof has enumerated categories of experiences that may arise in nonordinary states through breathwork as:

1. Sensory experiences and motor manifestations, which may include tightness, pain, numbness, tingling, temperature fluctuation, and even tetany.

2. Biographical experiences of events that have happened to us from birth to the present time, both positive and negative, releasing traumas of omission and commission and grieving. This reliving is more than just remembering.

3. Perinatal experiences from the fetal experiences during gestation and pregnancy, through the birth process, to the experiences immediately after birth.

4. Transpersonal experiences, which can take us beyond our bodies and our own personal (ego) identities. These could include conception, unity, out-of-body experiences, merging with other forms of life, becoming one with elements, other levels of existence, communication with an archetype, and yogic sleep states.[9]

Trainings for professional breathwork practitioners are steadily increasing in popularity as the potency and effectiveness of the technique is recognized and verified in clinical settings. Professional trainings are held in many parts of the world (see Appendix Two).

Personal Account

Lucas, a counselor, describes the profound experiences that can occur during nonordinary states of consciousness. These do not happen with every session, but when it does, it can lead to uncovering and releasing deep holding patterns.

"At first we did some very deep cleansing breathing. When pushed down, the lungs would surrender the little bit of oxygen it had stored for a rainy day. I decided this was the rainy day and pushed as hard as possible. Slowly the breath returned. It was quickly evicted from my body and just as quickly replaced; the session had begun. What seemed like several minutes passed with little to show. I still felt cold and uncomfortable, and the noise from the other breathers was disconcerting. 'Just keep breathing,' said my friend in the most reassuring voice. 'Trust that you will get what you most need at this moment.' With that I released my expectations of fireworks and watched my breath.

"It seemed as though I was breathing directly into my heart and it was opening. I could still feel the ground I was lying on, hear the other voyagers, and smell the scents around me, and still my consciousness moved away from ordinary.

"It was dark all around me, a terrifying and all too common sight. I had visited this place twice before—that too familiar scene of falling into a black hole, sides smooth as black ice, greased, and absolutely without footholds. I was dropping into a never-ending fall. After both previous visits, I had attempted suicide. I did not wish to pay a call to this address again. I kept breathing. Somehow my vantage point was raised and I was looking down on myself. Curled in a baby's form I was careening into eternal space. The ever-present loneliness made its appearance known. My heart, lungs, chest, and whole body felt like a vacuum cleaner had attacked. Nothing.

continues

"The cry that came from my body was chilling. Primordial, it must have rung true and shocked the facilitators for they were by my side instantly offering words of encouragement.

"Falling, crying, no hoping, lost. I was surprised at the feeling; it was the loneliness I felt at my parent's divorce. This was strange since the divorce had occurred many years earlier; I had already dealt with the issue. It was behind me. Yet here were the feelings bursting my chest in this moment. 'Please don't leave me. Don't leave me. I want you; I need you. Please.' It melted into an everlasting, full-body baby sob—the kind when toes, fingers, and earlobes get into the act. My body was shaking, and though I knew I would be all right, I experienced the fear of my past total annihilation. I felt I was falling forever as I wailed out. As each second passed, I wanted to stop this process. Yet I continued.

"Eventually, I landed back on the ground with a friend holding my hand and whispering comforting words. He had written down what I said, adding positive affirmations to remind me of my victory. I had made it through a fear I had run away from for years. It took another session to totally exorcise this demon, but this was the foundation. It showed me I could face death without destruction. I felt happy that I cried so fully; I had not done so since childhood. This work showed me that my mind could alter my surroundings when focused. It helped me trust my friends and, more importantly, the process."

Ethical Concerns

As with any new tool, breathwork can be used well or misused. Counseling opens participants to very vulnerable states. Adding the component of a nonordinary state of consciousness increases the necessity of clear ethical boundaries and competent training. Fortunately, several schools of breathwork have addressed this in the training of counselors.[10] An international alliance of breathwork schools and trainings have begun to create agreed-upon principles, ethics, and training standards for professional breathworkers.

The Global Professional Breathwork Alliance (GPBA; *breathworkalliance.com*) code of ethics delineates issues of client suitability, contracts with clients, practitioner competence, practitioner/client relationships, and practitioner interrelationships, as well as offering a set of practicing principles for breathworkers. The GPBA is also helping to set standards for professional breathwork training and has a list of resources for literature and research on its site (see Appendix One). The International Breathwork Foundation (*www.ibfnetwork.com*) is another source for information on affiliated breathwork centers worldwide as well as literature in several languages.

Differential diagnosis is also important in knowing what clients are appropriate for such intervention (e.g., clients who are not integrated enough to work with altered stated of consciousness or with whom the practitioner feels uncomfortable or outside of their scope of practice).[11] More peer-reviewed journals are needed to collate the growing body of research literature in this field (see Appendix Three).

Professionals from varied domains have used breathwork training to enhance their healing skills. Some of the disciplines incorporating breathwork include psychotherapists, occupational and physical therapists, nurses, physicians, dentists, massage therapists, and other body and energy workers. Each discipline must monitor the ethical use of the breathwork techniques according to its acceptable standards of practice.

Not every counselor is going to want to incorporate breathwork as an adjunct to his or her counseling practice. Nor will every counselor be attracted to use breathwork for her or his own well-being and self-care. This is as it should be in a pluralistic society. But every counselor and every client breathes; the commonality of breathing is a link that brings us all together. The breathing patterns of a counselor as well as a client tells a great deal about their moment-by-moment state of ease and resourcefulness in their lives. Breath awareness is a valuable adjunct to the healing arts even if formal breath modulation techniques are not employed. The growing field of breathwork is contributing valuable data to the conscious and therapeutic use of this simple yet powerful tool we all have right under our noses.

In the next chapter, you will learn about the principles of Therapeutic Breathwork and how they translate into formal sessions and community life.

Chapter 2

Principles of Therapeutic Breathwork Facilitation in Counseling and Community

This breath of life that breathes in each one of us is what one basically calls freedom. In biology it's called Life, in affectivity it's called Love, in psychology it's called Consciousness, and in theology it's called God. The difficulty is to bring these all together within everyone's understanding.

—ALFRED TOMATIS, MD

As you will see in the next chapter, the various forms of breathwork have grown with or have been applied to counseling and other healing modalities throughout the last century. The contemporary development of Therapeutic Breathwork in the latter part of the twentieth and early twenty-first century has been concurrent with a shift in consciousness from survival to an orientation toward growth. As such, its philosophical tenets reflect a more open system of values.

My home base has been in the Milwaukee, Wisconsin, area where, under the umbrella of Transformations Incorporated, I directed the School of Integrative Psychology and the Creative Consulting and Counseling Services from 1980 until 2013. Ours is just one example of Therapeutic Breathwork integrated into psychotherapy in the Midwest in the United States. There are several examples of such schools and counseling centers that are growing in strength throughout the country and the world. If a holistic orientation calls to you as a therapist or a client, then I encourage you to follow your heart and find the teaching and counseling that speaks to your soul. The advent of holism as a philosophical tenet in the latter part of the twentieth century heralded a fundamental shift in consciousness from linear or causal thinking toward systemic awareness. We can no longer operate with a mechanical model if we are to understand the interdimensional realities that allow us so much freedom and expansion of our capabilities. It is critical that we have a psychology that not only admits the existence of the human spirit but also takes it fully into account in knowing and predicting human behavior. Just as important is for us to have a notion of spirituality that incorporates the discoveries we have made about the mind-body connection and how the mind and body mirror and manifest our spiritual intentions. To keep these realms separate is to keep us split and severely limited in our understanding and treatment of the whole human being.

What Are the Principles of Contact and Contract Applied in a Therapeutic Breathwork Session?

These principles are designed as guidelines for anyone facilitating a breathwork session, which is a dyadic interchange in which one party guides another through a conscious, connected breathing cycle to help release holding patterns in the physical body, negative and limited belief systems, emotional constriction, and spiritual disconnection. *Contact* refers to how the breathworker connects energetically to the client. *Contract* refers to the conscious agreements between the breathworker and client as to what their exchange will be. These principles apply to almost any authentic human interaction in the helping professions.

Heart-Centered Contact

This approach views the client's emotional intelligence (EQ) as relevant if not more so in their healing and growth process than their intellectual intelligence (IQ). Clients are not generally drawn to Therapeutic Breathwork because of cognitive deficits, even though cognitive functions may well be improved as a by-product in the course of healing. It is the broken link between the intellectual reasoning and the physical behavior that is causing disruption in their lives that most often brings them to seek help. This is graphically reflected in the position of the limbic system, which regulates our emotional states in a picture of the whole brain and is in between the cerebral cortex, which is the seat of our higher thinking, and the brain stem, which is controlling basic body survival functions. Our blocked and repressed feelings get in the way of our behaving the way we think we should. These feelings are not the enemy; they are sources of wisdom that need to be integrated into purposeful and pleasurable living. They have keys to this integration that have not been recognized or applied effectively. These keys are often frozen in place through the mechanism of trauma, which we will explore in more depth in Chapter Four.

Establishing a trusting rapport with a client is the first step to a successful partnership in the dyadic process. I may have encyclopedic amounts of theory and technique at my disposal, but if I do not connect on a heart resonance level with my client, there is a major roadblock to the safety needed for the client to get past old defenses to make more resourceful life decisions. This does not mean I must just like my client. There may be aspects of my clients I do not like. Therefore, I must be able to distinguish between their personality and who they are essentially. This entails another critical tool for effective breathwork facilitation: holistic vision.

Holistic Vision

I believe we are ultimately all of one piece, but as long as we have minds, we tend to see the world in polarities. Even though these polarities are temporary fictions, some of them can be more useful than others on the road to integration. A tool I use to help clients and myself in having acceptance and compassion for seemingly incongruous parts of ourselves and ways of being and behaving is *holistic vision*. From this perspective we all have a personality and a spirit. The personality part of us is by definition limited in its view of reality and is consequently fear-based because it cannot see the whole picture and is unsure of its survival in the world. The more secure higher self's job is to help the personality navigate in the world and educate it to bring it increasingly into alignment with its higher purpose. At times it seems like the agendas of survival and purpose are at odds, and we become conflicted over decisions and besieged by feelings pulling us in opposite directions. Holistic vision is a point of view that allows us to see the "picket fence" of fear and doubt that our personality has erected for protection and also to see the essential being of love and peace that resides in the "inner house."

In seeing holistically, I can have compassion for others and not see them as just barred and defended or attacking, knowing that is not who they are essentially. But I can also have respect for and not trip over or be hurt by their defenses and fears. It gives me a better sense of when to draw closer or keep the distance they are asking for and not take it personally. I also become more proficient at detecting what part of me is in the forefront of my interactions. In other words, I can ask myself the question, "Am I hiding behind my defenses or inviting others into my home?" Awareness allows me to then make a conscious choice about what serves me best rather than playing out unconscious relationship patterns. I often sense my greatest gift as a breathworker-counselor is simply to hold the vision of my clients' essential wholeness and goodness even when they are in the depths of their fear and doubt. This does not create dependency on me for their well-being. I serve as a model for their practicing holistic vision with themselves. The more I practice applying this to myself, the easier it is to employ it with my clients. As a breathworker, being able to see with holistic vision is critical to not getting caught in my clients' fears but helping them to see them for what they are and breathe through them to the essential self they are seeking to affirm. If I notice that my defenses are triggered in working with a client, holistic vision helps me recognize and breathe through my fears, not letting them reinforce stuckness for myself or my client. Thus, a mutual healing is taking place synchronously.

Synchronicity

The concept of synchronicity is another vital tool for the breathworker. It is much more than a philosophical premise that there are always both personality and higher-self dynamics that are potentially healing for both client and practitioner in their work together. It is a daily occurrence for me that my clients will introduce issues that are "hot topics" in my life. My personality could either run for cover and try to avoid the topic, I could get enmeshed in giving them advice I myself do not follow, I could commiserate with them and reinforce our mutual stuckness, or I could turn the tables and try to get advice from them. Better than any of these personality-driven responses, recognizing synchronicity in play, I proceed knowing that if I give my best in both listening and sharing as well as continuing to breathe myself, more light will come both for my client and for me. At times I may judicially use self-disclosure, sharing part of my process with a client, but only doing so to the degree that it supports their process rather than downloading my emotional charge onto them. This takes radical self-honesty and lots of practice. The forgiving grace in synchronicity is that even if not all is cleared or released in a session, we are still connected, and the more I continue to do my work in healing, the more clients energetically receive the benefits from it on all levels if their spirits are open to it. Synchronicity takes the concepts of transference and countertransference of traditional psychotherapy to another level of responsibility. How the client projects qualities, traits, motives, and so on, on the therapist (transference) as a normal part of the counseling process to be used to help them see and deal more effectively with their past programing, as well as how the therapist may also engage in projection onto the client (countertransference), are a significant part of therapeutic awareness and responsibility in many, but not all, psychotherapy models. In addition to this awareness and mandate to take responsible action, especially if countertransference interferes with the client's healing process, the breathwork paradigm suggests that a mutuality of themes and healing is an inevitable part of human interaction. It is especially impinging on breathworkers to be attentive to their own healing process such that they do not confuse it with the client's process, unconsciously put it on the client to do the breathworker's work, or, in denying their own healing, slow down or interfere with the client's progress. Synchronicity is a foundational principle of a holistic systems model of universal interconnectedness, and, as such, awareness of it helps to raise the consciousness of both clients and practitioners in every encounter.

Personal Account

Lillie, a licensed clinical social worker, reports that awareness of the connection between her own breathing and anxiety has been a great asset in assisting her clients.

"As I was attempting to get to the airport and traffic was not cooperating, I notice anxiety and tightness in my chest and belly. Going to my breath allowed me to calm down and be in the moment.

"I was drawn to do breathwork in the early eighties after reading *Loving Relationships* by Sondra Ray. This began a connection with breathwork and my own awareness of my breathing and my body. My own breathwork has facilitated being in my body and being able to notice when I am not. I have cleared many negative beliefs, the bottom-line belief being 'I am unwanted.' My breath has brought me to a more loving relationship with myself, which continues to be a place of growth. I continue to claim more aliveness on all levels by working with my breath. It is my first go-to to become more aware and present.

"As a licensed clinical social worker, I notice and think about what people are doing with their breathing from our first meeting on. I give homework of full-belly breathing to do daily. This has lots of positive impact for people: decreasing anxiety, increasing the ability to fall asleep. I am often heard to say, 'Take a big breath.' Restricted breathing is common to almost everyone. Just working to open up clients' breathing changes a lot, increasing their ability to be more centered, more aware, and more connected to their body and emotions, helping release emotions rather than stuff them. The breath helps people hang out in feeling good, which is hard for many. We have been so acclimated to feeling less than that."

Multilevel Awareness

This concept of multilevel awareness is not referring to the levels of beliefs and values we will talk about in Chapter Three. The levels to which a breathworker does well to be aware of are states of consciousness that range from the subconscious, dream states, consensus reality, memories, and nonordinary states to higher consciousness. They are all in play for us all continuously. Our attention, though, rarely focuses on more than one or two at a time. In a breathwork session, awareness often becomes heightened, and several states may be activated in the same session (as referenced in Grof's list on page 7 in Chapter One). The breathworker as well as the client might enter (or at least be aware of) these states independently or together. The more thoroughly breathworkers can accept these states in themselves, the better they can be in helping their clients not only accept but benefit from these states. Messages, transmissions, insights, and epiphanies are all common to the process. How much of these are useful for the client to communicate to the breathworker and vice versa? Again, the breathworker's self-acceptance may be more important as a model, allowing the client to practice self-integration at times rather than reporting a breath-by-breath account to the breathworker after the session. A rule of thumb I use is to encourage only the amount of sharing that assists the validation and integration of the client. That also holds true for the breathworker's sharing with the client. In general, the client's sharing takes precedence, though there are times when the breathworker's process is very valuable to the client. Listening to one's inner guidance is necessary every step along the way.

Breathworkers from around the world have collaborated in putting together a list of principles for the "best practice" of breathwork compiled by the Global Professional Breathwork Alliance. They are a well-conceived compendium and are reprinted in Appendix One for reference.

Responsibility for Quality of Contact

Contact is the energetic interface between practitioner and client. The breathworker is responsible for the quality of his or her portion of that interface before, during, and after any formal sessions. As a breathworker, how I think and feel about my work sends an energetic message to the world and plays a part in whom I attract as clients. It can be sensed in my advertising, in my communication with clients before sessions, and in the general attitude I disseminate in the community about my work.

A breathworker's energetic quality may be oversolicitous, seductive, aloof, intimidating, or any number of ways that posture the breathworker toward the client and have an effect on the quality of the trust and the outcome of sessions. Because of the intensity of the process for the client, it is incumbent upon the breathworker to be clear, balanced, and boundaried in thoughts, feelings, words, and actions. This is not a dictate to be perfect or saintly in all spheres but to be as congruent as possible in our energetic messages. This is for the protection of the breathworker as well as the client. Breathworkers' unconsciousness about their energetic messages will be mirrored in their clients' process. Ultimately, if both are well intentioned and good-willed, there can be mutual healing and growth as a result. Our professional code, nonetheless, compels us to continually examine our own journeys and eliminate as much interference with our clients' healing process as possible. It has been noted that the nonordinary state of consciousness can heighten both the sensitivity and the vulnerability of clients. This is the reason for the call to a heightened sense of awareness, responsibility, and ethical boundaries that comes in Therapeutic Breathworker training. That responsibly does not coopt clients' responsibility for themselves and the results they achieve from their sessions. Indeed, as you will see in the "breathwork contract" in the next section, clients are given 100 percent responsibility for what they conclude about their work. But breathworkers also take 100 percent responsibility for what they give and receive from a session.

This responsibility for quality of contact applies to after a session is over as well. How breathworkers think and feel about their clients continues to energetically affect them. Again, "negative" thoughts and feelings may arise regarding clients, but it is breathworkers' responsibility to not harbor them or send negative energy toward their clients. Moreover, it is breathworkers' responsibility to "come clean" to themselves on their judgments and own the trigger and emotional charge within themselves that generates their judgments. It is not a requirement to like how every client presents him or herself but to have enough awareness not to project or harbor ill will toward them.

Contract-Agreements Between Practitioner and Client

The essence of Therapeutic Breathwork is learning a self-regulated skill for which the client must take personal responsibility for the outcome. The breathworker's responsibility is to teach this skill as best as possible, helping the client in on a journey of self-exploration and healing. As such, the breathworker is a breathing coach who educates and help guide clients in finding more conscious self-regulation. If breathwork is presented as something being "done to" the client by the breathworker whose skill is responsible for the client's healing, the result will be another disempowerment of the client and dependency upon an external authority.

The clients must know from the start that they are being coached to learn how to use their breath and intention to make positive changes in body and mind and to bring them more in alignment with their spirit, whether it is stated with these words and concepts or not. All of this can be conveyed under the model of health improvement if those terms are more fitting for the client (e.g., "I'll be teaching you effective breathing techniques that bring your physical, feeling, and thinking self into better alignment for leading a fulfilling and happy life. It is your job to apply these techniques to you in finding greater comfort and control of your life").

Depending on the profession of the breathworker, there is particular information they may want to know to better help the healing and growth process. For instance, if the breathworker is a physical therapist, they may want a more extensive physical history than a psychotherapist, who in turn may ask for a more detailed social and emotional history.

Breathwork per se does not require physical touch on the part of the practitioner. However, if a practitioner is a massage therapist, it may be a normal part of his or her practice. Information gathering and use of touch are all part of the contract between client and practitioner. Even though touch is part of my scope of practice as a therapist trained in Bioenergetics, I always ask permission of the client before attempting any intervention that entails touch. I have clients open their eyes, and I explain to them exactly what the intervention will entail (e.g., holding their feet for them to push against) and get their permission before making contact.

It is also good practice to explain that the breathing induces nonordinary states of consciousness but that the client will be aware of what takes place and will do only what they choose to do in the session. As with most professional codes, what transpires in the breathwork session is held in confidentiality by the breathworker, and any records of the session are also kept safe and confidential.

Delivery of the breathwork session is part of the practitioner's fulfillment of the contract. In sessions subsequent to the first, I always start the session with reaffirming the client's intention for the session, which also reminds clients of their responsibility in holding that intention. I get clear on my intention. Then we begin the process, following simple instructions on breathing with the willingness to let go and surrender to the process rather than trying to rigidly control it. I liken it to the control of a surfer learning to ride a wave versus the control of a dam trying to hold back the river. As a breathworker I have the willingness to step into another's world while staying grounded in my own and to go beyond my mind and also stay boundaried. I am both a teacher and a student, keeping balance in the process and seeing the client as both a mirror and a sacred companion in the cocreation of a new model of being whole relational beings.

Sessions vary in their intensity and aftermath. It is important to help client integrate their work after a session. I help them get grounded before leaving and communicate what is important for them without getting too analytical. I explain that it may take a while for all the material to settle into new awarenesses and life applications and to give themselves time and space to let themselves reintegrate after the session. I let them know my availability should they need to connect between sessions, even though that has been a rare occurrence. We plan a follow-up, and I often give them homework and resources in the interim. The homework may include reading the affirmations or "inner child" questions I write for them. I often introduce the concept of "inner child" to indicate their feelings as a child, which are still alive in their emotional body. Adults are often more willing to admit to their uncensored emotional state when it is put in terms of a "child" part of them. As they move closer to accepting this child part of themselves, they become more comfortable in accepting their feelings. The following are questions they might be encouraged to ask of themselves each day, along with other narrative work before or after they do some gentle connected breathing at home:

- "Where are you, little [their name as a child]?"
- "What do you feel?"
- "What do you need and want?"

I often suggest for "extra credit" they journal the responses to these questions and bring the journal with them to the next breathwork session. The simple childlike responses often give us clues about deeper feelings that their adult self may be willing to admit. They can develop the habit of awareness of the deeper feeling level using this metaphor of their inner child.

Clients often ask how many sessions are a normal part of the healing process. This depends on their goals, time, and resources, all of which I take into account in trying to help them get the most out of the session or sessions we do. Again, I emphasize that an important goal is their gaining the confidence in using both maintenance breathing and faster than normal breathwork as part of their normal life skills. Personal and professional goals are interrelated aspects of a holistic perspective. It is common that Therapeutic Breathwork clients make career shifts based on greater clarity and sense of personal purpose as well as confidence in achieving their life goals.

Transparency and accountability around payment for services helps keep the breathwork, safe, boundaried, and in integrity. I have made a training video entitled *An Introduction to Therapeutic Breathwork and Live Demonstration*[12] of a session as I conduct one. This is available at *www.transformationsusa.com*. It is not meant to be a template of how all sessions should be conducted. Indeed, no two sessions I have done are the same. It is intended to be an example of how a counselor or therapist might use breathwork with a client. I often intersperse breathwork sessions with talk sessions depending on the needs of the client. Even in the talk sessions I continue to be aware of the breathing we are doing together and will give feedback to my clients to help increase their awareness of when their breathing becomes restricted. The session in this video is relatively calm and integrating, fitting the client's needs at that time. A video demonstrating more activating sessions with techniques for the body themes covered in Chapter Five is also available at the above site.

Contraindications

There are two major areas of contraindication for doing Therapeutic Breathwork that have to do with the client's readiness and the breathworker's readiness for the work. Client readiness for Therapeutic Breathwork involves their sufficient knowledge of what the technique offers for them, their ability to integrate deep-level emotional and paradigm shifting work, and their willingness to engage. The breathworker must assess all three areas and be sufficiently convinced that these prerequisites are met to proceed with the session. Practitioners will present breathwork as they have integrated it into their professional skill set. A psychotherapist will have a different skill set and teach the principles of connected breathing as it relates to his or her approach to treatment differently than an occupational therapist, for example. The goals of how breathwork blends with why a client came to seek help from each respective profession will be different. The psychotherapist may stress how the opening of a client's feelings toward his or her mate during a breathing session can be translated into different behaviors in the relationship, whereas the occupational therapist may stress how the release of tension in the pelvic area after an injury can lead to different ways of carrying him or herself in a work setting. Both can have profound emotional and mental implications for the client's self-image and self-esteem but will be facilitated differently by each practitioner operating within the scope of his or her own professional training.

There is mounting research evidence for not only the safety of faster than normal breathing but also for its therapeutic efficacy. Some 11,000 psychiatric patients were exposed to holotropic breathwork sessions over a twelve-year period in a variety of clinical setting with "no nursing staff reports of untoward sequelae or complaints after the sessions during this twelve-year period," according to James Eyerman, MD (*http://metslesvoiles .org/wp-content/uploads/2013/12/HB.pdf*)

The second area of contraindication for Therapeutic Breathwork involves practitioners' readiness to take clients through the process given their comfort and expertise in dealing with the issues clients are seeking to resolve. The rule of thumb here is for practitioners to be honest with themselves in distinguishing therapeutic challenges that stretch them appropriately as a professional versus challenges that they are not ready to take on through lack of training or their own emotional readiness. In either of these cases, it is of utmost importance to make an appropriate referral so the client is not shamed or made to feel defective in not being treated by the referring practitioner. It is of great service and an integral part of the healing process to honor the client and practitioner relationship enough to make such a referral.

What Are the Core Values in Therapeutic Breathwork and How Does the Breathworker Live Them in the Broader Community?

Quoting Father Seraphim: Our life hangs only by a breath. It is the thread that links you to the Father, the Source, which brought you into being. Be conscious of this thread, and go where you will.

—JEAN-YVES LELOUP, *Compassion and Meditation: The Spiritual Dynamic between Buddhism and Christianity*

The basic training of a therapist or counselor coming to Therapeutic Breathwork has been directed toward helping clients get beyond reacting as victims of life circumstances. The scientific approach for professionals is to find behavioral and emotional patterns that lead to predictable dysfunctional results and to assist clients in redirecting these patterns. To have these changes be more than situational, it is necessary to uncover core belief structures that shape clients' realities. This, of course, is an art as well as a science, employing our intuition, empathy, and sense of timing as well as observational skills and theoretical approaches. The ineffable missing element, however, without which all the empathy, understanding, and technique will not suffice, is clients' *deeper sense of purpose*. The ability to inspire this is perhaps a Therapeutic Breathworker's greatest gift. However, it alone is not sufficient to bring a permanent shift in lifestyle.

To pretend that Therapeutic Breathworkers are neutral technicians of mental-health principles does an insidious disservice to clients and communities. It promotes the illusion of the value-free authority rather than that of the value-honest leadership. This highlights the potentially uncomfortable position that Therapeutic Breathworkers are in: our values affect those we treat and the community in which we live and serve. This is not only true when we are directly in the public view but also true in the more subtle standard we bear as the professionals who bring troubled community members into functional balance—for example, from politicians and CEOs in marital or legal trouble to the socially disenfranchised. Setting ourselves up as moral paragons or the "new religion" is rightly repugnant to all. But to deny our values and influence is equally irresponsible. How do we sort this out and ethically conduct a practice in such a pluralistic, multileveled society? Just keeping out of trouble by trying to stay safely within the limits of current codes of ethics is reactive and ultimately defenseless. What is an empowering proactive stance that does not require being a public crusader?

"Know thyself" is the pithy yet powerful rejoinder for all in helping professions. If Therapeutic Breathworkers know their values, they can responsibly communicate them and dialogue with their clients and community. This can result in an appropriate referral when their values are sufficiently different to be of disservice to their clients. It can also lead to more effective intervention in circumstances that are laden with conflicting societal realities. Therapeutic Breathworkers see "reality" as a medium for creating rather than a source of limitation, and it has four distinct levels. Translated into their work as therapists, they help their clients deal with the following:

- Challenging daily events
- Chronic patterns of behavior
- Underlying positive and negative belief systems
- Personal life purpose

Therapists who focus just on life events and patterns of behavior may heighten clients' awareness, but an inevitable frustration ensues for clients who can see their patterns and even predict their cycles but are unaware of the deeper structures that keep them in place. Therapists who are self-aware enough of their own belief systems are able to help clients unearth self-limiting mental models held in place by unresolved emotional and behavioral reactions. They then can help clients choose and transplant new foundational principles with the sensitivity of a gardener helping to tend to and celebrate new growth. As exciting as this may be for both therapists and clients, it too can lack the juice to inspire clients to self-direct and flourish. They know how to change but not why they are changing.

By having the courage to unearth and tap into their own purpose, Therapeutic Breathworkers cannot guarantee that their clients will (nor can they have them) feed off their purpose before they both burn out. They can, however, create the medium for clients to explore their own "whys" for living, help take their clients through their dark nights of the soul, and witness them emerge with their light in their time. This, of course, is truly rewarding and one of those perks that keep Therapeutic Breathworkers in practice. Even this ability to inspire can lead to disillusionment if we do not help clients go through all the stages of their own self-awareness, including a working mastery of their patterns and underlying beliefs. This means teaching the tools to self-search and championing their courage to challenge structures of fear and limitation as a lifelong mission. This requires an unflinching commitment to the truth and a willingness to challenge internal and external systems that inhibit taking full responsibility of their life and their membership in their community. It is not becoming a crusader or blind believer but rather a purposeful, connected student and teacher of meaningful life values. Therapeutic Breathworkers *deal with the why to live, not just the how to live.* This is not an intellectual process entailing the adoption of a belief system but an internal awakening to one's own life force and its connection to all of life. It does not prescribe any particular set of behaviors other than what promotes the growth in awareness and harmony in interconnectedness for all.

The outmoded arbitrary division relegating the whys to religion and the hows to science has long since shown its ineffectiveness and subsequent moral erosion. Therapeutic Breathworkers are called, I believe, to take the lead in admitting what they value, rather than being in denial and communicating unrealistic ideals (i.e., the illusion of the neutral human). Their ethical values may include respect for autonomy, nonmaleficence (avoiding harm), beneficence, justice, fidelity, and veracity. They must know and understand their values and be honest with the creative tension between that which they aspire toward and how they currently operate. This is a more realistic leadership model within our current world of advertising "hype" or cynical disbelief in anything. Ours is not to impose values or answers but to help an honest soul-searching inquiry into our purpose as humans living in an evolving, diverse, sometimes scary, yet creative world.

There are many examples of Therapeutic Breathwork being shared by holistic agencies and practitioners in communities throughout the world, but I can speak most accurately about the work I have done as an example of aspiring to the goals of Therapeutic Breathwork. It has been my life's work as a psychotherapist to investigate all forms of conscious growth personally and professionally. I examine and experiment with what others present from ancient traditions and new discoveries. I then retain those skills and practices that provided the most lasting, grounded results. This includes fitting the appropriate techniques to the student or client at the right time to facilitate her or his empowerment.

"Spiritual" for me signifies coming from the undefined spirit or animating force of life. "Religious" signifies a particular body of teaching or dogma about the origins of existence and/or living according to a proscribed moral standard. Some very "spiritual" (in my definition) students and clients have been atheist or agnostic. That is, they have a profound respect for the individual point of view and the sacredness of life itself. Other clients successfully journey with their traditional religion as a viable vehicle for their spiritual development. I was privileged to teach breathwork to the staff of an open-hearted Christian counseling center in the greater Chicago area.

Most clients come for personal healing and are at a transition point in their lives. They are looking for an environment to foster self-knowledge, forgiveness, and the joy of finding a path to their true heart's desire, rather than someone else's formula for a happy life. These are the clients who do well with Therapeutic Breathwork.

Not everyone is willing to take on this level of challenge, but those who commit themselves to a course of Therapeutic Breathwork have been almost universally grateful and permanently changed. If a holistic orientation calls to you as a therapist or a client, then follow your heart and find the teaching and counseling that speaks to your soul.

Personal Account

Rick is an ordained minister whose profound breathwork experiences were translated for him into spiritual terms that were most impactful for him.

"My most significant moment was during a breathwork session in water with Jim Morningstar. I remember relaxing into the warmth and support of the water. Fear came up for me with the sensation and I had the thought that I could not get enough air. I talked myself through the fear as I stayed with my breath.

"Soon, I felt compelled to leave the hot tub where I had been breathing. With Jim's help, I slowly crawled out of the water, keeping my eyes closed and staying with my breath. In my mind's eye, I had a vision of myself as a rapidly evolving amphibian, moving from a water home to a land home.

"Once on dry land, lying on my towel, I experienced a spiritual 'birthing' into the Universe. Still closing my eyes, I sat up and knelt, raising my hands and my voice to the sky with the words, 'Here I am! Here I Am!'

"Angels and guides fully supported me as I came into their world. They were celebrating me! At this revelation, I broke down and wept. Never before had I been so fully supported and received.

"In the next moment, I became aware of the presence of Jesus. He was standing before me, offering me a bite of bread to eat. What he was offering me was not only bread, it was his body, too, just like the script says in a church communion ritual.

"My first thought was, 'No, I can't. I don't want to cannibalize you. I don't want to diminish you.'

"Jesus's response was, 'You cannot diminish this body. I draw from a source that is everlasting. Eat and be filled.'

"So I did and I was. It was a wonderful experience of surrender, support, and fulfillment. I realized through this religious vision that all my fears around 'not having enough' are based on illusion. This experience allowed me to see past the illusion of lack to the true abundance and support available to me when I open myself to receive from a loving Universe."

In the next chapter, you will learn how the road to growth and emotional well-being has developed in our human history, particularly since the end of the nineteenth century.

Chapter 3

The Evolution of Therapy and Breathwork

While failure is possible, there is nothing that
Cannot be transmuted.
Our mistakes are our teachers and our alchemy
Is in our heart's blood.
Our breath is our point of entry to truth.
It is with us always, as us, as all of creation.
Find the breath in everything.

—DAE GAK, psychotherapist and Zen Master,
from *Upright with Poise and Grace*

The human nervous system is continually evolving and helping us adapt to and survive in changing environments. Degrees of complexity within the brain have given us continually increasing options in both adapting to and changing the world around us. Since the 1970s the National Institutes of Health and general systems theories have correlated a progressive series of cross-cultural developmental matrices.[13] What I present in this chapter is a condensed and greatly simplified overview of these levels of human neurological, cognitive, and consciousness growth taken from the work of Clare W. Graves, PhD,[14] and the roles that psychotherapy and breathwork play in it. This will put in a broader context the place that therapy and breathwork have for us now and in the probable future of our evolution, as well as to where the human need to help one another may be taking us.

Therapy involves the facilitation of change in the consciousness of the individual. From the levels point of view, this necessitates an assessment of the individual's present phenomenological state, the barriers the individual is encountering, and the direction in which the individual is heading, as well as a knowledge of the techniques that generally facilitate change at that individual's level of consciousness. This assessment is aided by an awareness of the individual's learning systems, past (child-rearing) and present, which will indicate the incentives and milieu most conducive to promoting change for the individual. This provides a basis from which to understand what stimuli are perceived as threatening, what coping mechanisms are used to maintain oneself, and what goals the individual is striving to attain. The sources for such information can be the individual's self-report, interview and test behavior (e.g., *The Way I See It*[15]), dreams and fantasies, and family or important others in one's environment.

"Ontology recapitulates phylogeny" is a way of saying that the growth of each individual reflects the growth of humanity over vast stretches of time that is built into our complex nervous system. As children we progress in a foreshortened way through the history of human civilization, systematically awakening growth in neurological complexity at each stage of our development. The progress of our inner neurological development is synchronous with our abilities to effectively interact with more and more of our environment (see Figure 1).

Letters *A* to *F* in the upcoming figures represent emerging neurological systems that, in combination with letters *N* to *U* representing the quality of one's external environment, result in markedly different existential states in our evolution (*A–N*, *B–O*, *C–P*, which will be described later). Thus, individuals do not evolve in a vacuum but in concert with changes in one's cultural, social, and physical environments.

Growth from functioning at one level of neurological and psychological complexity to another is not an instantaneous occurrence. It takes place over time at a rate that is often consonant with both genetic and environmental readiness. Every individual is a complex of potentials that are all operating and overlapping at any one time (see Figure 2).

Figure 1.

**Representation of Adult Personality as
a Complex of Bio-social Ecological Systems**

Conditions of Change

1. Biological equipment
2. Solution of existential problems (Readiness)
3. Dissonant stimuli (Impetus)
4. Insight
5. Overcome barriers

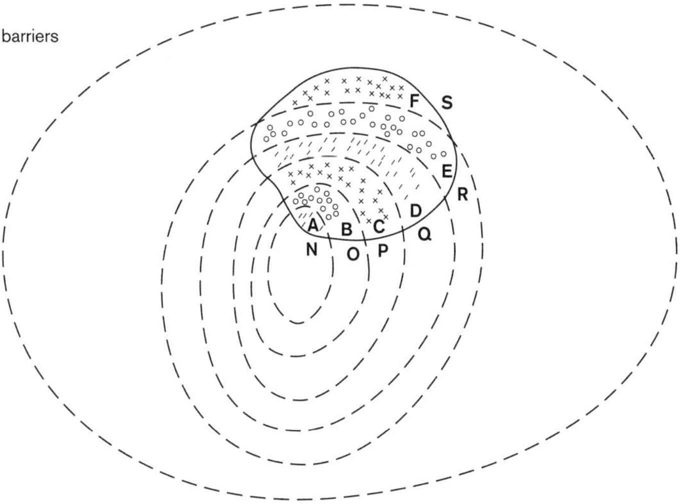

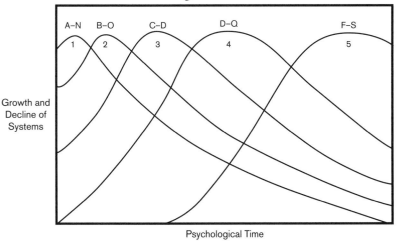

A–F = Different "dynamic neurological systems"
N–S = Qualitative variation in state of external affairs
A–N, B–O, etc. = Existential states
xxxx's, oooo's, ////s = Qualitative difference designations

Figure 2.

Growth and
Decline of
Systems

Psychological Time

We tend, however, to predominantly use one centralized nodal system until we gain competence in its functionality before we are able to incorporate the next. The fact that these systems have been charted does not establish a hierarchy of value or importance according to where one is in the developmental process, which in the end turns out to be more circular or spiral than a straight-line growth. People can lead happy, fulfilled lives or not at any stage of being. Truth, integrity, love, and the sustaining and transformative power of the breath operate at all levels and are especially needed to make successful transitions to another level. Open systems individuals will thrive more in seeking growth until they reach a satiation point when they become a more closed system and specialize in developing mastery at that level. Humanity seems to require all these levels operating at once, with individuals achieving states of peace, love, and joy at each level, for a unified field to be achieved and for humanity as a whole to evolve.

The themes and challenges for human evolution have been suggestively depicted in a series of diagrams from the 1970s from the visionary Clare Graves. The following are the themes for existence associated with each existential state:

Figure 3.

(from Clare W. Graves)

Theme for existence associated with each existential state:

1. A–N: React naturally to imperative physiological needs so as to reduce the tension of them. No concept of cause and effect.

2. B–O: Live in accordance with established tribal ways.

3. C–P: Express self for what self desires regardless of the consequences lest one feel ashamed.

4. O–Q: Sacrifice the desires of self now in order to get reward later or in some other realm.

5. E–R: Express self for what self desires but in a rational, calculating way without feeling shame or guilt.

6. F–S: Sacrifice what one desires now in order to get reward now in the form of acceptance by and approval of others.

7. G–T: Express self as self is inclined but not at the expense of others.

8. H–U: Sacrifice the idea that man will ever know what it is all about and go on living.

Problems of existence represented by each letter:

N   Achieving stability of imperative physiological systems.

O   Achieving basic safety in a not-comprehended world which seems full of spirits.

P   Awareness of existence as an individual; how to live against the fact of death.

Q   Reasonable order in a world of seeming chaos; how to live in a world of threat and want.

R   Reasoned knowledge leading to control of the physical universe; how to conquer threat and want.

S   Comprehension that human subjectivity is a reality, not a myth to be cast aside; how to live in a world of abundance for human wants.

T   Restoring ecological balance disturbed by the knowledge accrued; how to restore disturbed universe.

U   Truly accepting the reality of ever broadening realms of consciousness; how to live when having, but never really knowing life.

What was most amazing to me in reviewing this research was that decades of cross-cultural research confirmed that human consciousness growth takes place in an orderly manner from an "express self" system to an "adapt self" system to an express self system and so on, each stage building in complexity on the last. Whole groups of people tend to follow in this progression and grow together and share each other's values. In a complex culture, however, many levels coexist, and values can easily clash. According to Graves, a question like "What is the best way to educate children?" cannot be answered simply. More to the point we must ask, "What children, in what milieu, at what level of consciousness?"

As we grow, our neurology and environment synchronously grow and so do the educational and motivational models that will work best for us. The reason so many and diverse forms of therapy have come forth is that they grew out of the needs of certain people and environments at certain times in their development. No one model serves best for everyone. What you will see in this chapter is rather how more enduring principles of health and well-being have been adapted to evolving models. In particular, you will see how the breath, and its use, has been adapted to each level and can often serve to integrate the levels of development within individuals and among groups of people.

The first factor necessary for individual change from one level to the next is a basic organic *potential* for growth; a severely brain damaged individual is limited in capacity for conscious growth. Second is a *readiness* factor; the problem of existence must be adequately solved at our present level before we can maintain our existence at a higher level (e.g., at level two, "achieving basic safety in a not-comprehended world that seems full of spirits" in Figure 3). Third, there must be the *impetus* for change toward a more adequate form of existence, which entails the introduction of dissonance in the system at the proper time; this dissonance is different for each system (e.g., for a tribal level two individual to be exposed to a charismatic leader not adhering to tribal customs and surviving with greater freedom). Fourth, there must be *insight,* the acquiring of new ideas, for living that precipitates movement toward a new form of life (e.g., "How could I leave my tribe and form a new allegiance that is fulfilling?"). Fifth, the environmental impediments, or *barriers,* to movement must be overcome (e.g., safely leave the tribe with adequate provisions and join the new band without being killed).

"Mental illness," from this perspective, is viewed and treated differently from level to level. Symptoms are methods of coping that are fitted to the central psychology of a system. Anxiety and compulsive behavior are characteristics of even level systems (emphasis on adapting self), whereas acting out and impulsive behavior are associated more with odd level systems (emphasis on expressing self). A disorder may arise from a level other than the one at which a person is centralized; its treatment would utilize the principles of learning appropriate to the level from which the disorder arose. An example is a phobia, which often arises from the level-three system and responds to the principles of operant conditioning, even if the individual is centralized in a higher system.

Personality growth in a *vertical* direction comes with meeting all five factors for change; it results in the development to a higher level of consciousness (see Figure 4). *Oblique* change occurs when a base system takes on some higher-level characteristics; it is the result of solving only some of the thematic problems of a particular level while meeting all the other factors for change. *Horizontal* change produces a more complex form of a base system; this is caused by a lack of insight and/or potential for growth while satisfying the other factors for change (e.g., a level-five employee moving to a more humane corporate system while still embracing corporate values).

Figure 4.

Representation of Three Basic Forms of Change
Whem Higher Potential for Change Present

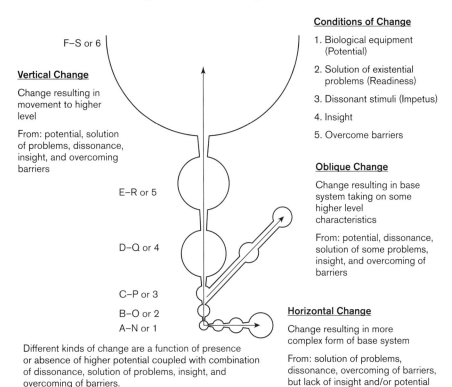

Conditions of Change

1. Biological equipment
   (Potential)

2. Solution of existential
   problems (Readiness)

3. Dissonant stimuli (Impetus)

4. Insight

5. Overcome barriers

F–S or 6

Vertical Change

Change resulting in
movement to higher
level

From: potential, solution
of problems, dissonance,
insight, and overcoming
barriers

E–R or 5

Oblique Change

Change resulting in base
system taking on some
higher level
characteristics

From: potential, dissonance,
solution of some problems,
insight, and overcoming of
barriers

D–Q or 4

C–P or 3

B–O or 2

A–N or 1

Horizontal Change

Change resulting in more
complex form of base system

From: solution of problems,
dissonance, overcoming of barriers,
but lack of insight and/or potential

Different kinds of change are a function of presence
or absence of higher potential coupled with combination
of dissonance, solution of problems, insight, and
overcoming of barriers.

Personality development is an epigenetic process in which each level of consciousness both grows from and expands upon a central core. Personality is an integration of all operative levels with the central or nodal level (see Figure 5). Although individuals tend to centralize their personality in the schema of one level, an open-systems person manifests many features of levels he or she has passed through as well as levels he or she is growing toward. A closed-systems person tends to eliminate features of any other level than his or her nodal level. An arrested-systems person shows the characteristics of an open-system individual, but any upward development is sharply curtailed by barriers. Personality growth in an open-systems person is most easily facilitated by individuals in the next higher system, whereas change in a closed-systems person is more readily facilitated by individuals within that person's nodal system. Thus, an open-systems client will respond well to a helper who has integrated higher-level principles. A closed-systems client will respond better to a helper who has more expertise within their nodal system. Individuals can promote change in people who centralize levels several steps lower, but they tend to become personally dissatisfied and find this work less fulfilling over an extended period than work with those closer to their level.

Figure 5.

Nesting Aspect of Adult Personality Systems

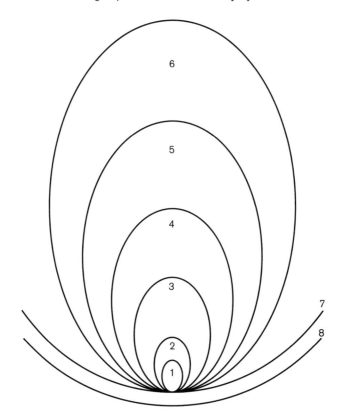

When new system takes over, lower level system is subordinated in the newer system.

When lower level system dominates that part of higher level system emerging operates in service of lower level system.

This is an example of a centralized level six system with developing level seven and eight systems.

Vertical growth in levels of consciousness involves transitions between levels, and these transitions follow a typical pattern. A point of value crisis is reached when the factors for change at any level are met. This often precipitates a sense of alienation and initiates a regressive phase. This phase is marked by behavioral turbulence and searching for a more adequate form of existence. During this regression, behavior may revert to that of the period of transition to the same family of systems (even level or odd level) immediately prior (see Figure 6).

Figure 6.

Progressive-Regressive Development of Symptoms

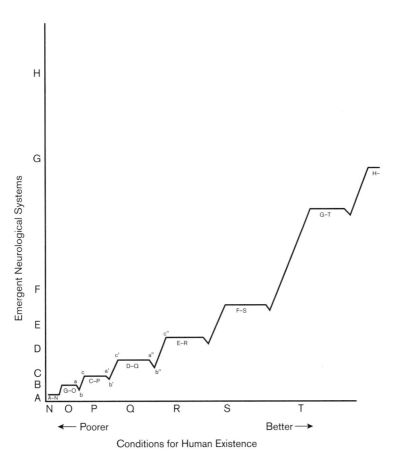

For example, an individual transitioning from level five to six (Pragmatic to Sociocentric) may revert to behavior patterns employed in transition from level three to four (Egocentric to Saintly). In looking for values that are less materialistic and competitive, express self (five), the individual seeks a system that values more sharing and cooperation, adapt self. So, the individual reverts to older forms of rules about behavioral conduct and submission to higher authority (Saintly, four). This does not, however, support the person's newly evolved individuality. It is not until finding a group of like-spirited individuals who value shared feelings, experiences, and mutual empowerment that the individual can adapt, but now it is to the will of the group rather than to a person in the seat of power. If he or she does not find this higher-order adapt-self community, a secondary regression may occur to a similar transition point prior to that of the primary regression. In the previous example, this would be to the transition from level one to two, searching out a more tribalistic form of existence. This regression continues until a point of behavioral crisis is reached, when the established forms that embody the prior way of life are confronted. At this time the insight into new forms of existence comes to the fore, and the barriers to them are overcome. For example, the individual finds others of similar values to whom they can relate and establish ways of life that support their values (see the earlier Figure 3).

People most often seek counseling during periods of transition when old definitions of self and safe structure are in chaos. Physiological as well as psychological changes mark such times and are evidenced in tension and deregulated breathing. At these times both slower and faster than normal breathing can be advantageous in facilitating new learning and reestablishing at least periods of homeostasis. How breathwork is introduced must be resonant to the belief systems through which the person is transitioning: level-three breathing to increase power and stamina, level-four breathing the right way the body was created, level-five breathing to effect peak performance, level-six breathing to feel good, level-seven breathing to harmonize internal systems with environment … and, of course, combinations of these as appropriate.

Each of the levels of consciousness will now be examined with regard to their basic problem for existence, physiological correlates, learning system, values, therapy, and forms of breathwork appropriate to developmental challenges and growth.

First Subsistence Level (Automatic Existence)

At the first subsistence level early humans are struggling to achieve stability of their basic physiological systems. Individuals here are simply aware of physiologically determined tension and its relief; behavior change takes place through habituation of built-in reflexological equipment. Little concept of self is present. The major problems encountered are those of primary survival, and the solution to these problems requires an environment in which survival needs are directly available to the organism. The organism adapts to the environmental conditions providing basic needs through the process of gravitating toward circumstances that promote satisfaction and away from those that portend danger. Learning does not take place consciously. Habituation occurs in all living systems and at all levels of a person's neurological hierarchy. Because humanity has on the whole evolved, level one is seldom seen today as a central system in groups of people except in rare instances or in individual pathological cases, any person operating at a higher level is always, in part, a physiological organism. Reactive values may come to the fore and dominate should basic needs be forsaken; an example is someone living on the street. When trauma to the organism is so severe that these basic organismic reflexes are inhibited (e.g., being hit by a bus), appropriate stimuli is required to be made directly available to the receptor organ to induce a resumption of automatic functioning (e.g., artificial respiration, intravenous feeding, heart massage). This is perhaps one of the most immediate forms of help to sustain the conscious life of a human, giving direct assistance to basic organismic integrity. Help with the breath here may involve direct CPR, intubation, and automatic ventilation.

Personal Account

As the author of this book, the following is my personal account of my father's introduction to breathwork.

"A life-altering experience for me happened when I was informed that my father, who was then in his early sixties, suffered a massive heart attack and was unconscious in the hospital. After three days of him being

continues

unconscious, I went to his bedside and whispered in his ear that he was loved and could come back if he chose and gave him some breathing instructions. Within a minute his heart monitor alerted the hospital staff to come immediately. He woke up during the next day and underwent triple bypass surgery. He had no conscious recall of my whispering to him but to my surprise agreed to do a breathing session with me a week after his release from the hospital. During this session his body mimicked all the symptoms of a heart attack. Images of headlines reading "Breathworker Kills Father" flitted through my imagination, but faith in the process prevailed. He felt no pain but reported feeling he had been given a new life. He lived twenty years longer, remarried after my mother died, traveled, and enjoyed many of the experiences he never had in his prior sixty years."

Assuming organic potential is present, growth to the next level of human existence can be facilitated when two conditions are simultaneously met. First, organisms acquire a set of conditioned reflexes that provide automatically and dependably for the continuation of their existence; second, organisms find that particular environment appropriate to the acquired conditioned behavior.

Second Subsistence Level (Tribalistic Existence)

A human at the second subsistence level is striving to achieve basic safety in a world that seems full of spirits. In this world there is no separation between subject and object, phenomena possess no clear contours, and things have no particular identity. One form of being can be transmuted into another; there is correspondence between all things. The concept of linear causality is not fully used; the individual perceives forces at work in life to be inherent in all things—human consciousness is linked at the deepest level. Time is seasonally based, and space is perceived in atomistic fashion. A society based on this form of existence is steeped in myth and tradition; being is a mystical phenomenon full of spirits, magic, and superstition. The individual has no existence apart from the tribe. Here the task of existence is simply to continue what it seems has enabled "my tribe to be."

The area of the human nervous system that functions most prominently at this level of existence is the brain stem, including the reticular activation system. This area takes a primary role in amplifying, regulating, and integrating all impulses passing between the higher brain centers and the body, and it regulates the autonomic reactions including all the vital functions of breathing, heartbeat, circulation, digestion, and so on. This neurological system is activated by changes, particularly sudden changes, in the mode or intensity of stimuli associated with one of the individual's innate reflexive networks, like a dog reacting to the smell of food or the odor of an aggressor. When this system dominates, learning occurs through the classical conditioning method; that is when there is a very short time between an arousal state and something to satisfy that arousal, like when an infant is hungry and presented with the breast. In humans this system dominates during the first month of life. Subsequently, it becomes subordinated to progressively higher and more complex nerve networks. When moderately stimulated, this system produces a transient orienting reaction leading to exploratory responses and ended by familiarity with the stimulus object. More intense activation produces an initial defensive reaction, followed by innate or acquired fear reactions, and terminated either by escape from the arousing stimuli or by habituation to a level-inducing exploration. The feeling of a threat to "basic safety" can arise by any stimuli linked with continued arousal of this system. In situations where the environment fails to provide any adequate support for the subsequent focusing of the defensive reaction, continued intense reticular activation could lead to the generalized irritability or diffuse anxiety that characterizes certain neurotic syndromes.

In a sense, all therapy entails some conditioning procedures, inasmuch as the individual associates new stimuli or absence of old stimuli with basic organismic safety. When basic autonomic reactions dominate the behavior pattern and there tends to be little reversibility to other levels of functioning, such as specific goal-directed behavior (sex, eating, drinking) or cognitively patterned behavior, a classical conditioning technique is indicated as the most efficient form of helping. An example of this technique is a tubercular patient who became addicted to medically administered morphine. He was successfully treated for the addiction by pairing a positive nonaddicting stimulus (rubbing the forearm) with gradually decreasing amounts of morphine. This patient did not choose the addiction for some higher-level conflict resolution, but his body had associated the absence of the drugged state with autonomic irregularity. The helping principle of most classical conditioning therapy is to reverse the original traumatic learned response or to desensitize the chronic anxiety state. This is accomplished by associating, in a gradually increasing hierarchy, the presence of the anxiety-provoking stimulus with a state of basic safety. This state may be induced through a relaxation technique or a previously learned, strongly rewarding response. It is practically impossible in the adult human organism to separate the functioning of the brain stem from other neurological systems. Most therapies that employ a classical conditioning theory (e.g., Wolpe, Salter, Jacobson) utilize other levels of functioning in the implementation of their technique. In line with the contentions of these theorists, it can be hypothesized that many symptoms that seemingly first arise at higher levels (e.g., relationship issues leading to divorce) may derive their energy from lower centers (early abandonment) and that the focus of this bound energy may come to be located there, making them much more amenable to the techniques that deal directly at the lower levels (physical contact and comforting). This appears to be borne out in some cases and is perhaps due to the primary sensitization of the organism during early development to the set of stimuli that is again encountered in higher-level conflict (e.g., separation, lack of nurturance).

Working directly with the internal wiring of primary fear responses to psychological issues has found more current success with techniques such as eye movement desensitization and reprocessing therapy and energy psychology techniques (e.g., tapping acupuncture points while associating positive self-acceptance phrases).[16,17]

Therapeutic Breathwork can facilitate change in classically conditioned fear or anxiety responses that were preverbal by pairing the arousal state (activated by faster breathing) in a safe and supportive environment that gradually desensitizes high arousal through conscious, connected breathing. The individual is literally reconditioned with coaching when anxiety sets in to breathe in a self-regulating way. Talking about these states with clients may give temporary reduction of arousal but pairs this satisfaction with the consulting room and the therapist. This creates a classically conditioned dependency that may take years to generalize outside of the therapy setting. Therapeutic Breathwork pairs the learned satisfaction with the quality of breathing itself, which is more easily transferred to the client's life outside the consulting room.

Personal Account

Dana, a massage therapist, is a highly talented and intuitive healer for others who has struggled with her own anxiety and obsessive compulsive issues that talk therapy did not resolve. She shares her experience in her own words.

"Breathwork has helped me get into a more open, relaxed, safe space to share and process during therapy. Breathwork combined with therapy has helped me uncover patterns and beliefs from childhood and early adulthood causing problems in the present. The breathwork enables me to stay with these feelings/emotions and process them in a safe and deeper way. Specific techniques have helped me release long-held anger, fears, and frustrations. In addition, it has given me tools to use in daily life to cope with anxiety, OCD, and depression. Breathwork and therapy helped me form a deeper, more meaningful connection to Spirit and my Higher Self, which to me is invaluable, and I am extremely grateful."

Facilitation of growth to the next level of existence requires that sufficient and consistent rewards be provided to conditioned responses such that a surplus of energy arises in the individual with which he or she is able to explore the environment beyond the bounds of his or her safe tribal existence (which in today's world is simulated by the family) and realize his or her individuality vis-à-vis the world. People who recognize their individuality and have the ability to shape the environment to fulfill their needs outside of the prescribed traditional ways, yet who are similar enough to others such that they can identify with like drive states in themselves, are good facilitators for this transition (e.g., the heroic figure).

Third Subsistence Level (Egocentric Existence)

In the egocentric level of consciousness, humans become aware of their existence as individuals pitted against the forces of the world and faced with the threat of death. For the individual at this level, "might makes right," and existence depends on a controlled relationship between those who have the ability to seize and retain power and those who are forced to submit. This is referred to historically as the Attila the Hun level and developmentally as "the terrible twos."

Concomitant with the awareness of self and survival based on the satisfaction of individual needs is the emergence of the operations of the subcortical forebrain including the thalamus, hypothalamus, and limbic system. This network, which begins to mature during the second month of life, provides (1) more refined sensory discrimination and motor coordination, (2) specific motivational and/or emotional orientations supporting ongoing behavior sequences, and (3) mechanisms for the control of attention. Characteristic of behavior at this level is that it seems to arise from internal sources (i.e., drive states) and be directed toward stimulus patterns associated with consummatory activity (e.g., sex, eating).

Humans learn at this level from those bodily movements they produce that bring satiation of a specific drive state. That is rewarding, which provides them with their survival needs of food, water, sexual satisfaction, and the secondary rewards closely associated with these. In this trial and error or instrumental learning scheme, reward is dependent on the organism's active behavior. The degree to which learning takes place is a function of the amount of activity spent getting to the reward, the length of time between the desired consummatory activity, the presentation of the reward, and the strength of the need state. Immediate gratification is of high value here.

Deep and persistent behavior patterns are associated with the satiation of these major drive states. It is during this critical period when the objects of emotional significance are determined. Although myriad social and moral behaviors mediated by higher cognitive patterns surround the satisfaction of these needs, associations on the operant level often run counter to and are more compelling than logical or moral convictions. Conflict at this level can paralyze any part of the organism, as in a hysterical conversion reaction, immobilize functioning in a particular setting, as in phobias, or precipitate stereotyped compulsive behavior that only partially satisfies some basic need but is kept from completion by an equally strong repression. Therapy with conflict problems at this level comes under the broad rubric of behavior modification. An example is Skinner's technique of shaping, which involves rewarding closer and closer approximations to any desired behavior. Applied in reverse to eliminate an undesirable behavior (e.g., a phobic response to snakes), the individual is rewarded for a favored response in closer and closer approximations to the stimulus situation, which elicits the behavior to be eliminated (e.g., staying inside for fear of encountering a snake). Another technique for eliminating an undesired behavior is to associate an aversive response to the stimulus situation, which brings gratifying but unwanted behavior (e.g., a medication that causes nausea when alcohol is consumed). People dealing within this level of existence, such as native Africans, have used these techniques for centuries. In our culture, a cure for enuresis in the male child can be accomplished through using a bed pad with an electric grid in it attached to an alarm that rings loudly (aversive stimulus) when the child urinates (undesired behavior). The child is rudely awakened at each wetting and often eliminates this behavior. The Africans accomplish this by tying to the enuretic's penis a frog that croaks loudly (aversive stimulus) when the child urinates during the night, also often bringing an end to the enuretic problem.

The therapeutic process for conflict at this level requires a setting controlled to the extent that an appropriate drive state can be elicited and direct reward (through as many sense modalities as possible) and immediate reward (one to three seconds after the behavior is emitted) can be consistently administered. When a complex behavior such as speech is being taught, the operant process must begin at the level on which the individual can respond and increase in increments no larger than can be integrated. This is standard behavior modification procedure.

In a Therapeutic Breathwork session the client is first coached to associate a connected breathing rhythm with safety (safe supportive environment and facilitator—classical conditioning). As the work continues, the client then learns to self-initiate the connected breathing rhythm through whatever sensations, emotions, or thoughts arise during the activated state (operant conditioning).

Their internal drive state toward satiation (release of tension, pleasurable flow of energy, heightened awareness, and sense of joy) is paired with self-initiated regulated breathing. In Therapeutic Breathwork clients are instructed to connect their inhale to their exhale without pause in a slightly faster rhythm than a resting state. This initiates an activated sympathetic system. They are further instructed to balance or self-regulate this rhythm to sustain it to release and resultant homeostasis. What it takes to do this is different for every individual; everyone learns by their own trial and error what leads to release and pleasure for them. They are directed to assume responsibility for their healing from the start. This increases confidence and self-esteem as self-soothing is mastered in more and more life situations.

Personal Account

Debra is a high-energy author and Reiki master who was shaken to her core when her sister-in-law, with whom she was very close, was killed while riding her bicycle by a drunk driver. Anxiety, grief, and pain curtailed her functioning physically as well as psychologically. She also developed a phobia of bicycle riding. Breathwork helped her release her bound fear and pain and learn self-soothing on the noncognitive level. She even overcame her bike-riding phobia.

"For me, Therapeutic Breathwork was the modality that gave my body the healing it needed. I had been in physical pain for about a year, after the sudden and tragic death of a family member. I had been unable to grieve, and the more I suppressed my feelings, the greater the pain in my body became.

During that year of pain I went to many doctors; I received Reiki, massage, physical therapy, and acupuncture; and while all of those treatments helped, the pain endured. It wasn't until I received Therapeutic Breathwork that my healing began in earnest, and the pain began to diminish.

"I liked the combination of talk therapy and breathing. Feeling safe with my therapist I was able to start talking about how I felt, something I desperately needed to do. This loosened me up, and after an hour or so of talk I would lie down and breathe.

continues

"The breathing took me to a place of altered consciousness, which took me out of my head and allowed my body to do what it needed to do. I was able to release not only my grief but also many years (and lifetimes) of unhealthy thoughts, emotions, and feelings that had been stuck in my body. It was a big release, and it really allowed me to get out of my own way and let go. After a session I always felt lighter and liberated. After a year or so of monthly sessions, the pain in my body was gone, and I was able to access my feelings and openly express my grief.

"While I no longer receive Therapeutic Breathwork, I enjoy monthly group breathwork sessions, which continues the process and allows me to heal on all levels—mentally, physically, spiritually, and emotionally. I am very grateful for this modality and its powerful healing abilities."

Growth to the next level requires individuals to be presented with a system of behavior in which they can channel their drive states to ensure reward in the form of more cognitive signs (sublimate), even when the direct environmental rewards appear lacking (delayed gratification). Strong individuals who exude power and authority yet who have learned to control their drives and whose fear has been displaced to a power beyond physical force (that "higher power" that controls the universe) are good facilitators; their power must be recognized by those whom they wish to help, and they must show themselves as not submitting to drive states or the power ethic, while recognizing their existence (e.g., the transition from an Attila the Hun style of leadership, which is level three, to a Mahatma Gandhi style of leadership, which is level four).

Fourth Subsistence Level (Saintly Existence)

Establishing reasonable order in a world of seeming chaos is the problem facing humans at the fourth level of existence. Humans strive to learn how to live in a world of threat and want. They attempt this principally through finding the rules and prescriptions of that higher order according to which ones the world and their self must submit. Inner peace and ultimate salvation come through avoiding any opposition to this order and suppressing and repressing their inner drives, as well as from a strict ordering of the outer world. These are necessary for achieving harmony with this order. Rules are black and white, and only one authority is supreme.

At this level there seems to be a more coordinated functioning between the brain stem and subcortical forebrain and the introduction of neocortical input into the patterning of behavior. Another physiological development at this level is a relative abundance of adrenalin in the system, making the individual particularly attuned to aversive stimulation (punishment).

Abundance of adrenalin makes the avoidance of punishment a powerful motivating factor. In this avoidance two-step learning there seems to be a first stage in which a stimulus is associated with pain (classical conditioning) and a second stage in which a specified response averts the pain (operant conditioning), although this latter response is often complex enough to suggest higher cortical input. Here, avoiding what is punishing is learned first, and reward comes later in conforming to that behavior that successfully averts punishment. When this state is central, no punishment seems to mean no learning, too much punishment produces rigid and most difficult to change learning, and wrong punishment seems to leave the person unaffected or to produce negative hostile learning. This system (two-factor learning) is quite ineffective, however, when applied to the impulsive, anger-prone, immediate-reward-seeking individual of the previous level. Taking a child living in survival off the streets, setting them at a desk, and telling them if they do not wiggle for a week they will get gold star does not produce the desired results no matter how many times you hit them with a ruler ("saintly level" pedagogy).

Therapy within level four (the "saintly system") entails more than simple insight. When the values of this level have been violated by giving in to the impulses to immediate drive gratification (sin) of the previous level, a state of anticipated punishment ensues. The tension (guilt) is not released until punishment follows (penance), and the "correct" response is strengthened by a positive motivation and action (expiation). Communication of the tension state to another consciousness (confession) is often an important step in this process. Attempts to "strengthen motivation to do right" is a therapeutic aim that has existed for ages. This approach has been incorporated into formal therapies and programs like Alcoholics Anonymous, which take guilt, confession, and expiation seriously and involve twelve steps of action rather than mere "groping for insight," as their proponents have admonished.

Clients may seek breathwork from some degree of level four motivation; for example, an authority figure said it would be good for them. An ability to delay gratification for a later reward is necessary to go through the therapy process (i.e., enduring the sometimes uncomfortable sensations and feelings that come with breakthrough processes). But staying with the process over time takes more personal responsibility than just "I'm supposed to do this because I was told it is good for me." Clients must experience the reward as resulting from their desire to release and courage to breathe in the face of their fears. The nonordinary states of consciousness that can happen in breathwork have facilitated breakthroughs from fear and guilt states that are translated in religious and/or spiritual terms and become quite motivational for people. (See the account of Rick, minister, in Chapter Two.)

Personal Account

Julieann, foster parent trainer and mother of a developmentally disabled adopted daughter, was profoundly shaken when her daughter drowned. No amount of intellectual consolation removed the grief, guilt, and disillusionment with God that she suffered.

"Lily was my precious daughter who died from drowning when she was only eight years old. She came to me during a breathwork session with Dr. Morningstar. During the breathwork experience, I was about eight years old. I was distraught and crying that nobody cared I was hurt or that I felt sad. Nobody comforted me, and I felt alone. This represented my true childhood memories. Then Lily and angels showed me that they came to me when I was that crying child. They shared their knowing that I deserved to be comforted, and they were with me then, comforting me. Lily also let me know that is why she came to me physically as my daughter.

continues

"This breathwork experience helped ease my grief in a way that just talking about her from my memories could not have done. I understood and reaffirmed my belief that life is eternal. Her being, her spirit, existed before she was born to this life as my daughter Lily, and it continues still in the nonphysical where she continues to love and care about me. Interacting with Lily in this loving, nurturing way after she passed away was a wondrous experience I will always treasure."

Facilitation of change to the next level requires that an accepted authority introduce some dissonance into the individual's learned pattern while they are in a protected environment (e.g., the consultation room), that is, where they are not subject to punishment from previous critical authorities.

To promote this growth to the next level, the opportunity for individual decision-making and reward-seeking must also be introduced. Dr. Freud, in the protected environment of his office, allowed his patients' punitive inner authorities to be challenged, admitting into consciousness impulses that would bring rebuke in their original settings (through "free" association). His patients tended to be mostly in transition from Victorian level four to turn-of-the-century pragmatic level five, which is more cognitively oriented; his task was to promote insight and curtail "acting out." Thus, his therapy utilized little of the action-oriented expiation of level four. His formulation of psychic mechanisms included an *id* or source of basic organismic energies that work on the pleasure principle of immediate gratification; this *id* encompasses many of the functions of the specific drives toward the animal satisfaction expressed in level three. The *superego* functions to keep the individual from "doing wrong" and is subject to all the hazards of rigidity and over-punitiveness of the learning mechanisms in level four. The ego exercises rational control of the individual and, in vacuo, is the pure ideal of level five (Ayn Rand's philosophy[18]). What is observed is that Freud's[19] psychic mechanisms correspond in function closely to the emerging levels of consciousness herein described at a critical point in the evolution of human consciousness and the development of higher-level neurological functioning. He was engaged in devising the methods to free up the emotional energies bound up in lower levels through incomplete learning or trauma and repressed or suppressed through the learning mechanisms of a level four punitive culture. Once lost level three objects (e.g., mother) were recovered to awareness, the emotion bound in formerly thwarted drive states could be expressed (catharsis) without the fear of level four censure. This energy was then available to the ego for productive rational work. The methods Freud devised (i.e., free association, dream analysis) bring the (level three) objects of immediate gratification into awareness, and many of the forbidden (by level four) emotions attached to them transfer to the therapist (stimulus generalization, transference), who through an accepting attitude helps associate a positive reward to their appropriate expression (sublimation). After this energy is released toward specific objects, the feelings of safety and a positive effect have to be "worked through" (generalized) to the rest of the patient's significant others and life situations that formerly reminded the patient of the forbidden stimuli. Freud's theory is an example of how different helping processes can be viewed in the light of emerging consciousness levels. Theorists, of course, are multileveled individuals, and their theories are likely to encompass several levels. Their practice, on the other hand, is likely to be selective toward methods that facilitate the movement of a clientele at particular levels of consciousness in the population being treated. This does not rule out the combination of methods as long as the principles of the client's centralized level of consciousness are not violated. Orne,[20] for example, combines analysis with hypnosis, which aids relaxation of lower centers. Jung[21] combined analysis with a higher-level experiential approach aimed at releasing creative potential.

Adler[22] took another step toward the next "express self" system in postulating a will to individual power as central to the human psyche. He further analyzed and exposed lifestyle patterns in an endeavor to facilitate the development of more efficient patterns, emphasizing the cognitive over emotional elements of human behavior. Rank[23] went further in sanctioning personal decision-making by allowing patients to determine when their therapy should end. These facilitators were dealing with a clientele heavily burdened with the repressive, punitive learning of the level four system (culture), and each developed theories of personality and therapies that reflected these problems of existence. As successful facilitators at this level they were authoritative figures; yet they were permissive within limits that would not overly threaten but rather encourage the independence of their clients. Their "authority" was that of their individual reasoning capacities, which paralleled the emergence of greater prefrontal cortex involvement in rationally directing limbic system impulses and controls.

Many of the same principles apply in Therapeutic Breathwork when dealing with issues at the client's fourth level of consciousness. The breathworker represents an authority figure onto which many primal feelings may get projected (needs for father or mother's love and approval). This is especially heightened during a nonordinary state of consciousness in which the client is vulnerable and suggestible. The role of breathworkers is to facilitate awareness of the client's needs, disengaging the old sources they were conditioned to seek (i.e., their parents or significant other's approval) while not transferring the object of these to the breathworker but rather the client's inner resources. Obviously a degree of self-awareness and healthy boundaries are needed by the breathworker to facilitate individuation for the client.

Personal Account

Jennifer, educational volunteer and a devoted mother of two daughters, one adopted, still carried with her the scars of her mother's suicide. The loss of that parent figure and lack of childhood guidance set her on a course of lifelong therapies that did not fully empower her. She used her positive transference in breathwork as a model to self-empower on an organic level, which has blossomed into ownership of her own authority (inner parent).

"I have always been someone who believes in therapy as a way to understand myself more and get insight into the challenges in my life. Over the last dozen years, I experienced what appeared to be trauma after trauma, coupled with an already shaky foundation from a difficult childhood. Despite my best efforts and those of numerous counselors over the years, the talk-based therapy I was seeking was not fully working for me. It was not until finding Jim four years ago, who introduced breathwork into our work together, that I have truly found hope and the ability to break away from what I thought was a hopelessly stuck place.

continues

"Breathwork has allowed me to experience myself in a whole new way. It has allowed me to detach from the part of me that wants to analyze my way out of all my problems and move into the part of me that can feel and know that I am OK, creating a deep and profound trust in myself. It has furthered a sense of love, support, and guidance that is within me at all times, even during periods of sadness, anger, and fear. I have benefited from having a therapist who himself is walking the same path. He knows that the type of change I am seeking is possible, and as a therapist who has and continues to do this work himself, he has tremendous insight into the true possibilities for all people who are hurting and feel little hope. Breathwork in the course of my therapy has allowed me to experience my inner world first hand, and with Jim or other breathworkers at my side, it has given me much greater awareness of my deeper feelings, my connections with others in this life, and a profound sense of peace within myself. I also believe that breathwork has given Jim more insight into my inner experiences and how I process what is happening in my life, which has benefited our work together tremendously, even in subsequent sessions in which no breathwork has taken place.

"One of the greatest benefits of breathwork for me has been that this work is truly transferable to all areas of my life. What I love the most has been the ability to parent my children in a way that takes their whole being into account and honors the fact that they each have their own inner worlds that are important for them to tend to. I now have tools and skills I am able to pass down to them that, I believe, allow them to live with greater compassion and love for themselves and others. I am forever grateful to Jim and all my teachers in their various forms, my children included, for opening me up to how beautiful life is, even during its difficult moments. Breathwork has been a profound key to this understanding."

Fifth Subsistence Level (Materialistic Existence)

How to conquer threat and want, how to control the physical universe through reasoned knowledge, is the problem of individuals at the fifth subsistence level. The mechanistic, measuring quantitative method is their main approach to these problems. They value gamesmanship, competition, the entrepreneurial attitude, efficiency, work simplification, the calculated risk, scientific scheming, and manipulation. This pragmatic, scientific, utilitarianism is the dominant mode of existence in the United States today (although a major shift to the next, sociocentric level, is well underway as Graves predicted in the 1960s).

At this level, establishment of more highly developed perceptual, cognitive, and motor capacities of the neocortex provides for awareness of patterns, giving ideational control to conscious experience and allowing more complex exploratory behavior. There is less direct internal press for immediate primary gratification, and "perceptual novelty" itself becomes rewarding. Through continuous activation of lower centers, the neocortical system is able to sustain long-term motivation in environments lacking constant reward.

Increased neocortical development allows learning to take place in other than immediate reward situations. The variety and availability of environments to exploration at this stage have bearings on later learning capacity, although the effects of deprivation are more reversible than at earlier levels. The latent or signal learning, which takes place here, is again an active learning method, as in the previous odd level system, but it is not as aggressive or demanding of immediate reward as the operant model. At this level the patterning of stimulation, changing and challenging ideational content, and the degree to which outcomes meet the person's expectations are the major motivating factors. Here individuals can wait for delayed reward if it is under their own control, not micromanaged by those in positions of authority, and replete with perceptual novelty. This learning does not have to be tied to a specific need state nor is it dependent on the amount of consummatory activity or immediate reward. The keystones are the opportunity to learn through one's own efforts, the presence of mild risk, the individual's experience, and much variety in the learning experience (see the work of E. C. Tolman[24] and J. B. Rotter[25]).

At this level humans are trying to increase the control of their behavior through the use of reason; they begin to see their problems in living as stemming from many interrelated factors. Sullivan[26] gave heed to the continued influence of interpersonal relations on an individual's characteristic patterns of living. His task as a therapist was to help elucidate these patterns for the client both through extensively examining previous patterns in their social history and through unraveling the meaning of the client's communications in the interview.

Therapy here is oriented toward freeing up dysfunctional patterns in living through unblocking the individual's cognitive organizing abilities, that is, helping the individual recognize self-defeating patterns and reorganize them in a more functional manner. Kelly[27] has devised a therapeutic process based on the understanding of the individual's "personal constructs"; he contends that all behavior is logical if the premises of the individual are understood. Again, the task is to help the client perceive the deficiencies in his or her constructs and try alternative planned roles. The Ellis[28] method of rational psychotherapy is another example of an approach that works efficiently with level five conflicts. Ellis attempts to correct neurotic misconceptions about life through unmasking the clients' illogical thinking of self-defeating verbalizations by 1) bringing them into the client's consciousness, 2) showing them how they contribute to their disturbance and unhappiness, 3) demonstrating exactly what the illogical links in their internalized sentences are, and 4) teaching how to rethink and reverbalize these and other similar sentences in a logical, self-helping way. Much counseling with individuals at this level takes the form of "exploration of resources" and "pointing out alternatives" for the clients in such a way that they understand that the responsibility for the actual decision-making lies with them.

Interest in broader life patterns also becomes evident in the helping process at this level. Social concepts take prominence over Freudian biology in the analytic therapy of Meyer,[29] Horney,[30] Erikson,[31] and Fromm,[32] to mention a few. Working with groups and patterns of group interaction also becomes more feasible. Although level four group therapies were devised, their leadership and direction are necessarily of a different kind. This holds true for artificial groupings of people or natural groupings (family therapy), in restricted locations (hospital milieu therapy) or in the community. The closer to level five the group participants are, the more they will respond to facilitative skill and the less they will seek authoritative power. Leadership here requires the ability to avoid individual side-taking, advice giving, or judging right and wrong, and requires the skill to grasp interactive patterns, point them out in a manner that will not introduce too much cognitive dissonance, stimulate the initiative to devise alternative patterns, and leave the responsibility for change with the individuals involved.

Certain theorists (e.g., Satir[33], Jackson[34]) have paid much attention to communication patterns in detecting conflict areas; Bateson[35] has pointed out the grossly discordant communication patterns in the families of psychotics. These patterns often contain conflicting messages from different levels in the sender and bring about a resultant tension in the receiver; for example, when a mother sends her child seductive "take me" (level three) cues with her body, while giving a censuring "thou shall not touch" (level four) message with her words, or when a father demands complete submission to his moral authority (level four) yet pushes for aggressiveness and initiative in getting ahead (level five), the resulting conflict may render all or part of those systems in the child inoperative (e.g., lack of appetite, bizarre nonconforming behavior, illogical thinking). The conflict may further cause a flight to other levels of consciousness (psychosis), an opting out of their stressful environment. Their environment, in turn, seldom provides support for functioning at those levels; hence, "psychotics" are often removed to a hospital setting where the stress is reduced and their skills in handling their "normal" environment are reinforced. When the nodal system of the conflicted individual is level five, intervention at the cognitive level required for communication theory is appropriate.

Personal Account

Mark, educator/librarian, has highly evolved intellectual skills and was challenged to "understand" the deep-seated patterns within him that caused profound turmoil. Combining systems-oriented talk therapy with breathwork along with seminars and readings was the best combination of head/heart work for him.

"Jim has integrated knowledge and practices from many disciplines into the work he does as counselor and teacher. One of the most powerful practices he uses involves our breath. Back in the day we called it 'rebirthing.' Since then other names have come and gone, but the central principle, that our breathing can be used for therapy and healing, has remained an important part of his work with us.

"In counseling with Jim, in our classes, and on our weekends, breathwork helped me 'get out of my head.' I could feel things in important ways that I couldn't always by talking about them. One of my early "rebirthings"

continues

helped me release a particularly virulent self-criticism and experience a transcendent understanding of who I am. A few years after that, the breathwork helped me understand emotional patterns in my life that seemed to have begun even before I was born. Many of my experiences with Jim and breathwork all by themselves would have changed my life. Combined with all the other work we did—counseling, yearlong classes, body-work, group-work, reading, writing, affirmations, weekends—the breathwork supercharged the transformations I was seeking. This work we have done together, which included breathwork as a central modality, has helped me be a healthier and happier human being."

Promotion of growth, the sixth level of consciousness, requires that the individual be in an environment in which the problems of material existence pose little threat. Both internal and external resources are sufficient to provide for basic needs as well as comforts, and the individual is brought into contact with others for whom sharing the benefits of existence is more important than acquiring them. At this transition there is a shift in emphasis from the patterns and process of life to the subjective content of individual experience. The focus in interpersonal relations is less on making them more efficient for supplying individual needs and more on bringing individuals closer to one another for gaining acceptance. Working in groups is especially indicated during this transition. Breaking down expectations placed on self and others that keep individuals from sharing on an equal basis is the task of certain Gestalt techniques.[36] Being aware of how one affects others and gaining the ability to communicate how they affect oneself is one of the major functions of sensitivity training.[37] "Consciousness raising" groups help to break the pattern of society that keep individuals segmented from each other; Bioenergetics[38] and structural integration (Rolf[39]) help to break the musculature patterns of the body that function to inhibit sensations.[40] Marijuana and mind-expanding drugs have been employed for similar effects especially during this transition. During the regressive phase of the transition, many earlier forms of subsistence (e.g., pioneer existence) are explored, and formerly rejected belief systems (e.g., Pentecostal religion) can be taken up. But the individuals in this transition bring to these older forms broader perspective and different consciousness of life than those in transition from level three to level four; these individuals often go on to create their own (level six) forms of life.

Breathwork in groups has been particularly effective in helping this transition. A popular form uses loud music to help induce nonordinary states along with the altered breathing rhythm; it's called Holotropic Breathwork, pioneered by Stan Grof, MD,[41] who also did early groundbreaking research on LSD therapy. Here the facilitators are instructed to be nonintrusive and nondirective in their approach to intervention.

Individuals involved in promoting growth at this level must be fairly well in touch with their own bodies, free enough from status or authority concerns to treat others as equals yet recognize their own abilities, and able to communicate their awareness of self and others in a medium of personal warmth and acceptance (e.g., Stan Grof).

Sixth Subsistence Level (Sociocentric Existence)

At this sixth subsistence level humans are striving to learn how to live in a world of abundance for human wants. They have the comprehension that human subjectivity is a reality, not a myth to be cast aside, and they direct their energies toward knowing their inner self and other selves so harmony and acceptance can come to be. The authority they recognize is that of their peer group, rejecting differential classification and espousing the democratic approach. Warm social intercourse and personal sensitivity are highly valued.

The functioning at this level seems to reflect a more refined integration between lower appetitive centers and higher cognitive processes. The learning system associated with this level has been variously called the vicarious, the modeling, or the observational learning system. Within this system individuals acquire new potential behaviors without receiving any direct external reinforcement for their own acts or making the observed response. The learning takes place through observing events or symbols, or the consequences of others' actions, without having to take a direct physical part in the environmental manipulation.

Helping at the sociocentric level is effective with many of the group techniques mentioned as useful in the five to six transition. There is a greater emphasis, however, on equality of participation and less of a therapist-client orientation. Each is expected to participate in the process of working out their own problems. There is a general dislike of specific formal techniques and a gravitation toward informal, empathetic sharing. Spontaneous interaction is preferred to a planned program or even fixed roles. Spiritual values are prominent, and again, as with previous even level systems, encouragement to uphold the systemic principles (e.g., equality, tenderness) is often the means of handling conflict arising within this level; but here the group provides the learning standard rather than an authority figure (level four) or an outside expert (level five).

Both individual and group breathwork help individuals at the sixth level explore their inner world of sensations and emotions and to free their flow. The ability to communicate with "emotional intelligence" or nonviolent communication (NVC) is highly valued at this stage of growth where sensitivity is equally if not more important than knowledge.

Breathwork helps develop a "felt sense" for individuals who have lived life primarily "in their heads." Here feelings are not judged right or wrong. They are sources of information that lead to life's richness. The breathworker helps the client to breathe with all feelings, including rage and terror, to recover the energy frozen in their suppression by trusting their breath and, where useful, directing the expression of these feelings to safe targets. This relieves great stores of anxiety for those who fear the "demons" within them—which turn out when exposed to be feelings that we were taught would cause loss or even "eternal damnation" if expressed.

Personal Account

Mike, computer-systems analyst, makes a good living being analytical but wanted to get out of his head into his feelings. Breathwork in a group setting was the impetus to breakthrough for him. He now not only participates in but leads some politically active groups in his community aimed at bringing differing points of view into cooperative efforts.

continues

"This was my first experience of breathwork. My therapist, Dan, had recommended it when I had asked for something more experimental I could do to further my growth.

"We did the session in the large room where the group had its meetings. I tried my best to do as I was told. My breath was now pretty quick, in the chest; it was no doubt forced, mechanical. I had never really thought about breathing before, so I was just trying to do a lot of it as I'd been instructed. For a while I just kept at it, wondering what could be the point, what I was supposed to be experiencing.

"So I moved around. I tried sitting up. I moved my arms. I could feel the energy run up and down my arms and into my shoulders as I raised it. I moved like a *T'ai Chi* practitioner, because it felt like a good way to let the energy flow in me. I had to move, lying down and keeping breathing as I'd been told was too scary. This was how I made the situation safe. Others in the room were making noise. A man was shouting 'F__k you, dad!' or some such thing—and I wasn't at all sure I was doing it 'right.' But I was so relieved to feel that my body was capable of this experience, of conducting this electric, liquid sensation from my contorted fingers down my arms, into my body, to the floor.

"Before this experience I had feared that my mind would never let me find myself. I'm not very in touch with my emotions, often, even now. And this session did not seem to have a lot of emotional content. But it proved to me, conclusively, that I have a feeling body. I knew that this energy I felt could be my ticket to a living encounter with emotion that that I'd feared would always hide behind my mind's filter.

"The main change in me from this experience was gratitude and optimism that I could experience myself so fully. It made a big impact on me how simple the technique was. "All I did was breathe a bit," I kept thinking.

That first breathwork opened the door to all the work I've done at the School of Integrative Psychology since then. Even if it hadn't, I would still have this diamond of knowledge—there is more to me than I notice most of the time, and I can experience it without anything more complicated than my own breathing."

Growth to the next level of existence involves crossing the chasm between sustenance and being, between deficiency and growth motivation. At this stage of transition the environment is providing all the sustenance needs of the individual who has learned to live in harmony with other valued beings. Growth to the first being level entails the realization of *all* beings as of ultimate value. Humans here begin to identify with all life. Overcoming the blocks to this is a task that the individual consciousness must undertake alone, for it is in realizing that each block is of one's own creation that the individual consciousness allows its greater identity to emerge. That is not to say that growth cannot be facilitated by another but that the major direction and initiative will stem from assuming individual responsibility. Facilitation is a process of helping individuals see the barriers to their growth, recognize the mental categories and attitudes they maintain, experience the emotions and sensations of their body, and reflect them back to the individual with as little editing as possible. This reflection helps clients to clarify their perceptions, feelings, and attitudes so that they come to be less identified with and blocked by them and are free to experience a broader identification with life. Rogers's[42] method of nondirective therapy approaches this helping model. An individual who is relatively self-actualized and who is clear enough of major neurotic response patterns to adequately reflect rather than edit may facilitate such growth (e.g., Abraham Maslow[43]).

Breathwork is particularly suited to this transition to what Graves termed the "being level" because it on the one hand addresses the physical, emotional, and mental energy blockages at the six substance levels, while on the other hand opens the door to the expanding consciousness of more global awareness. As Ken Wilber[44] points out, transcendent experiences are possible at each level, but they will be interpreted through the belief systems of that level. One may describe a religious experience while the other relates contact with cosmic consciousness. But for both it helps them transcend holding patterns felt as stuckness and to experience more flow and joy in their lives. With the help of a facilitator, this can go beyond just a transitory event to a freeing and employment of energies into more healthful and rewarding lifestyles. The breath serves as a continual reminder of this potential to transcend blockages and the power to consciously shift energy states and alter thinking patterns. Once learned, its potential for further growth is vast. Stage one in a breathwork journey is the clearing of dysfunctional survival patterns. Stage two is the discovery and exploration of the extraordinary potentials of the human being.

First Being Level (Cognitive Existence)

At the seventh level of existence or first being level, humans turn their attention to the problem of restoring a disturbed universe. They see how human knowledge to this point has often served to disrupt the ecological balance. They become concerned with developing an ethic based on a knowledge of cosmic reality, not merely human's egocentric desires. They now seek to restore harmony and perpetuate existence for its own sake. To accomplish this they set out to develop their powers of truly recognizing the magnificence of existence. They develop a genuine acceptance for the way things are and let their behavior be guided by that which will promote growth in each particular situation. They have a more truly detached point of view rather than the "objectivity" of the level five, which was colored by unconscious survival needs. They recognize the interdependence of all beings and affix less attachment to any one mode of existence or set of values. Their faith is in the unfolding of being rather than in any one means by which this is brought about.

Learning at this level takes place through a whole-person apprehension of each situation. More than the acquisition of intellectual information, learning at this level takes on the experiential qualities of realization with one's "entire being." The integration of lower and higher centers that began in level six is brought to a point of integration such that the systems involved in these centers appear to operate more as a total unit or Gestalt. Individuals take in the whole situation with their full complement of abilities working as *one* far greater than the sum of their individual parts. Learning here is particularized to each set of circumstances. If the situation calls for authoritarianism, then an authoritarian response ensures; if the situation calls for democracy, then a democratic response follows. This is seen as quite inconsistent by lower-level standards, but a level seven person is able to encompass all the lower systems and integrate their functioning into a much broader plan while remaining in integrity. An analogy of such integration may be taken from the practice of advanced *T'ai Chi*. This art allows individuals to be alert to organismic danger, mobilize bodily energies to defense, avoid harm to themselves, assess an aggressor's pattern of attack, and direct their energies in such a manner that the aggressor, even in an attack, is not injured. When accomplished with yielding compassion, level seven individuals respond with their entire beings to promote the harmony of existence.

To this point, level seven has been described as an ideal. Individuals here, as in every level before, have acquired emotional trauma, neurotic response patterns, and blocks to the free release of energies at every step along their development. Helping to overcome these barriers at this level, however, takes on a new dimension—the dimension of more integrated consciousness that encompasses and transcends the separate functioning of all lower systems. In the therapeutic setting, each barrier can be brought into full consciousness such that the instinctual, emotional, or cognitive conflict that a barrier masks is experienced with the entire being, not just by certain neurological systems. The more complete the conflict can be experienced and communicated, the more prone defense systems are to being dispensed with, the more body posture and manner of breathing are subject to transformation, and the more likely neurotic response patterns are to become outmoded. The task of achieving this full experience can be facilitated by someone who has an openness to contacting the client's consciousness in a direct open and accepting way. If the facilitator is free enough not to react in a stereotyped fashion, clients are more able to contact directly their bound energies. When this contact is complete, the defenses being set aside, it precipitates a release of energies bound in all lower systems. The reception of this release by the facilitator provides the completion of a previously thwarted attempt to contact the environment and is a necessary element in the release. Elimination of neurotic (incomplete looping) attempts to con-tact leaves an individual in a state of openness to life and ready for a more complete identification with all existence in the next level.

A supportive environment during this process is crucial. Facilitators can help to point out defenses or direct individuals to avoided areas, but their greatest asset is the ability to openly accept the conflicted, often emotionally laden, energies of the client. Unless the facilitator's directions come from an openness to the client, they will be perceived as the facilitator's own defenses and become another barrier to the client. The therapy medium, in other words, is clear consciousness and unconditional positive regard, not any particular counseling technique.

Therapeutic Breathwork, facilitated by breathworkers who have done their own internal work, provides a medium for clients ready for higher-level integration, to tap into areas of bound energy, whether through trauma or suppression, with an open systems approach. Breathworkers help set the stage for release by the openness of their own system. They provide a framework intellectually and emotionally for the client to explore deeper states, and they give the tools to activate their systems appropriately. When the clients' ener-gies are released, the breathworkers help them integrate and ground them during and after the session as well as offering tools for integration between sessions. The interactive presence of the breathworker becomes more than a model of integration; it is a magnetic force field that interacts with that of the client in a healing dance that will be further elucidated in other chapters.

It is easier to release energies bound in high-level systems and is pro-gressively harder to change patterns the more directly they are associated with basic organismic safety. Phenomenologically, ideas are easier to change than emotions, which are easier than sensations, which are easier than instincts. Conflicts at one level tend to have repercussions on all the levels built upon it; even if these conflicts become relatively isolated from the functioning at higher levels, they drain off tremendous reserves of energy in the effort to maintain that isolation and thereby deplete the energy avail-able at higher levels. The beauty of Therapeutic Breathwork is its ability to work on the most primal levels as well as the most expanded.

Personal Account

Lillie is a psychotherapist and certified Therapeutic Breathworker. Here she recounts experiences in her personal sessions that span from the most "primitive" and animistic to the most expanded and universal.

"It is not easy to pick one significant breathwork session from all the significant ones I have had. There is the breathwork session in which I saw myself as a child playing with the infant Jesus and then being carried on the shoulder of a man with crowds cheering and it turned into the baby Jesus. From this I came to realize I was not alone and that I had the perfect spiritual partner. Then there is the session when I became a buffalo snorting and pawing the ground.

"The wet breathwork I'm most drawn to write about at this moment is finding the inside of my heart. I have little recall of my time in the water. As I hit the mat outside the tub I became this huge red-orange beating heart. The strength, rhythm, and beauty mesmerized me. I wanted to suspend time totally and stay in this state of bliss in my heart. I felt awed by the wonder and beauty I found here. This heart so strong and so full of aliveness and love. Tears flowed gently from my eyes as I beheld this wonder, my heart. Never before had I known my heart. This experience gave me more awareness of the depth of love, depth of feeling, beauty, and strength contained within me. This experience has helped me live more and more from my heart. To listen and speak from my heart. My life is a Journey of the Heart."

Little is known about the transition to the eighth level of existence. Enough of the individual's life energies must be freed from neurotic survival attachments to their own ideas and devices in order to experience a more direct communion with being. An environment that sustains the individual, yet aids in breaking down mental sets acquired in the subsistence state, helps promote the transition. Meditation and mindfulness are used by some to help de-identify from subsistence sets. Through these methods and others aimed at confronting one's attachment to subsistence identifications, these identifications can often be released for brief periods. Unless individuals' internal and external environments are clear enough to maintain a steady state of "being consciousness," however, they soon revert to old patterns, often with their faith shaken in themselves, former defenses weakened, and an experience of profound existential anxiety. Some who are unable to integrate necessary lower functioning into a higher consciousness state, yet who cannot return to lower system identifications, are left in a nonfunctional, disregulated condition. Individuals at a higher level (some mystics and shamans) are reputed to be able to facilitate the growth of others through direct conscious contact, requiring no words or thoughts. This seems to entail a conscious act of opening up and letting the fullness of being flow through them to another whom they perceive as ready to receive the experience.

Second Being Level (Experientialistic Existence)

Having freed potential for growth and directed new perspective and insight into restoring a disturbed universe, humans reach the stage where they truly realize that there is much they will never know about existence. They come to accept the reality of ever-broadening realms of consciousness and forsake the task of "knowing" life in a strictly intellectual way. They enter a new form of existence in which the major value is not one of problem-solving but one of expanding consciousness. Their values are experientialistic, and their goal is one of communion with the fullness of being. Eighth-level individuals seek to increase their consciousness through opening themselves to the continual flow of being. They are not primarily concerned with manipulation of being as experienced at subsistence levels, but rather by manifesting authentic self, striving to become a vehicle through which others can overcome exclusive identification with lower system life.

There is a complete transformation of human physiology at this level of existence, characterized by a marked decrease in the autonomic indices of continual vigilance (readiness for fight or flight), i.e., lowering of blood pressure, increase in skin resistance, and so on. This is associated with a state of relative organismic security and lessening of everyday anxiety. The type of thinking at this level is called differentialistic. The individual is open to the totality of each experience and is not made anxious by seeming contradictions; they are all assimilated into the gradual unfolding of the universe of which they are a part. The more they manifest being in each experience, the more they increase the consciousness of the universe. Everything, then, is a potential "learning experience" when human consciousness is allowed to merge with it; when the exchange of consciousness is mutual and complete, there is a consequent increase in the energies of both.

Therapy at this level could be defined as any process that aids the individual to remain open to the flow of being. This includes subjecting any and all body and mental barriers to the "witnessing" of consciousness, many of which could entail pain and suffering because of their deeply rooted nature. The removal of barriers to experiencing the greater self usually comes easier than the removal of those that keep a person from the full experience of others or eventually all of life. Another conscious, open individual may help by receiving the experiences of the person trying to overcome barriers. If the receiver can remain open, he or she merges with and *is* that part of the sender that is willing to become conscious of hidden of painful areas. The more conscious the facilitators, the more willing and able they are to expand the consciousness of the client, because they have gone through those areas and no longer need to defend themselves (and others) from them. This process is directed toward the eradication of all identification with static identities or roles. This is living more consistently with *holistic vision*.

Breathwork provides the opportunities for clients to explore being in innumerable nonordinary ways. As cited earlier, one of Stan Grof's[45] categories of these experiences that have happened cross-culturally by breathwork clients is transpersonal experiences. These can take us beyond our bodies and our own personal (ego) identities to experiences of conception, unity, out-of-body states, merging with other forms of life, becoming one with elements, past lives, communication with an archetype, and Yogic sleep state.

Breathwork provides a doorway to exploration of high levels of consciousness in a safe atmosphere. It is a platform for continued human exploration and evolution.

Transition to higher levels of being can be depicted only through the consciousness of those on the leading edge of human existence. Some characterize the experiences of these levels in spiritual symbolism, calling the stage above the experience of infinite power, knowledge, and bliss, the stage of living both as human and the divine simultaneously. In this higher level, the person supposedly not only experiences but directly uses these realizations to the betterment of all life. These speculations take us into undreamed-of realms and await the fulfillment of consciousness manifest through us all.

This brief sketch of therapy and breathwork as seen from the levels of existence point of view is by no means complete or final; it is here to stimulate conscious thought about the process of helping. One of the contentions of this chapter is that humans can help fellow humans to survive, and grow and this process entails being able to meet others where they are at in life. Meeting others has been delineated in terms of understanding the problems of existence with which they are coping, what they value, how they learn and what motivates them, how they breathe and what frees their breathing and increases their energy levels, what seems to help them when they are in conflict, and what tends to promote the growth or realization of their consciousness. All the techniques proposed to facilitate the helping process are ancillary to basic empathy and compassion for fellow beings. Using this scheme requires the ability to recognize differences in conscious states and approaches to them while retaining the humility to recognize the infinite "godhood" in each. When the helper is too ego-involved in the helping or when the validation of one technique or dogma takes precedence over the give and take of the helping process, the mutual exchange of energies required for growth is short-circuited. Levels of consciousness are presented as an aid to reaching others rather than as a method of categorizing for the sake of holding them at bay; they are, of course, a temporary fiction, for all consciousness is in process and is ultimately one. In this proposed chain of being, each can increase the consciousness of another; each is both growing toward a higher level and elevating a lower level (albeit apparent standstill or regression). Every time someone is helped through a barrier to increased consciousness, the energies of both the helper and the receiver are increased and the total consciousness of the universe is expanded—part of the spirit that holds this book together is the faith that this is what we are about.

Personal Account

Mary Jo, a gifted healer, breathworker, and psychic, used breath and intention to heal her body and now shares the use of breath with those who come to her for healing.

"The marriage between breath and intention is a practice; no, rather a way of living. I have witnessed the power and grace of the breath plus intention in my life: scoliosis straightens, an arthritic finger unwinds, anxiety departs, the inner child recovers, the soul retrieves aspects to gain wholeness, fear disappears into nothingness, and so much more. The breath was instrumental in my journey of healing from crippling rheumatoid arthritis. Now in excellent health, I utilize the breath coupled with intention to create ease, joy, and flow in my life. I am thriving.

"This is my practice: Connect to the breath of life and know there is something more than just the bones, flesh, and blood of you. Be aware, concentrating on the in-breath touching the out-breath in the dance of life. Now just breathe, coupling breath with intention. Intention is your choice. Will it be healing, compassion, forgiveness, love, or thankfulness? Will this intention be general or specific? It's your choice. Easily couple the intention with the breath. Now just breathe. Now know, breathing is being."

Occurrences in the lives of individuals that lead to traumatic responses of chronic holding patterns or "freezing" provide some of the most formidable challenges to human growth and evolution. Trauma likewise presents some of the greatest challenges to those in the helping professions trying to assist their clients to higher integration. Here is where Therapeutic Breathwork contributes a vital link in the healing process. This is the topic of the next chapter.

Chapter 4

Therapeutic Breathwork and the Healing of Trauma

Controlled deep breathing helps the body to transform the air we breathe into energy. The stream of energized air produced by properly executed and controlled deep breathing produces a current of inner energy which radiates throughout the entire body and can be channeled to the body areas that need it the most, on demand.

—NANCY ZI, author, voice teacher

This chapter presents the role that trauma plays in our development on all levels and highlights the importance and usefulness of breathwork in healing the effects of trauma. The goal is to help you engage in exercises and learn techniques that you can safely and effectively employ when working with trauma in a healing session. My hope is to assist you in breathing clarity and passion into your life and the lives of those with whom you work.

An Overview of Trauma

This section defines trauma and discusses its causes, symptoms, and biological nature. It also covers memory's role in trauma.

Definition of Trauma

Major trauma can have a profound impact on a person's life, but as you will see, the physiological dynamics of the trauma process are experienced by everyone to some degree or another. Severe trauma can result from a stressful occurrence. On the physical level, Peter Levine[46] states, "The heart of the matter lies in being able to recognize that trauma represents animal instinct gone awry." If someone is overwhelmed by a threat and is unable to successfully defend him or herself (i.e., respond from their instinctual nature), they can become stuck in survival mode. This highly aroused state is intended solely to enable short-term defensive action. Left untreated over time, it can form the symptoms of trauma. When an individual is unable to flow through trauma and complete instinctive responses, these incomplete actions often undermine his or her life. It is not the event that is traumatic; it is the individual's perception of and capacity or incapacity to respond to the event. *Trauma is the frozen, undischarged energy held in the body and the mind that is often associated with feelings of defeat and helplessness.* Though we all can experience the effects of trauma, less than 20 percent of the population is predisposed to respond to severe stress in a highly traumatized manner. Dan Siegel suggests, based on the study of Attachment Disorders,[47] that early chaotic or terrifying exposure to a major parenting figure may be a significant factor in this predisposition. Nonetheless, not everyone who is exposed to the same extreme circumstances will develop the severe symptoms of trauma. Those who are more vulnerable to severe trauma will take longer to recover, especially if they have little support in the recovery process.

The causes, symptoms, and biological nature of trauma in the next section are based on the work of Peter Levine.

Causes of Trauma

The causes of trauma can be divided into two main categories: events that are most frequently traumatic and common, jarring, unexpected events that can be traumatic under certain circumstances.

The first category includes the obvious causes of trauma, such as the following:

- War
- Severe childhood abuse
- Experiencing or witnessing violence

- Rape
- Assault
- Catastrophic injuries and illnesses
- Loss of a loved one

The second category includes seemingly ordinary events that traumatize more often than you might expect. The following are some of these potentially traumatizing occurrences that may not be so obvious:

- Minor automobile accidents
- Invasive medical and dental procedures, particularly when performed on children who are restrained or anesthetized (even adults who rationally know that they are helpful may experience certain procedures as an attack)
- Circumcision (sociological research reveals the most warring nations medically and religiously promote circumcision)
- Falls and other so-called minor injuries
- Natural disasters
- Illnesses, especially high fevers
- Accidental poisoning
- Abandonment
- Prolonged immobilization, especially for children
- Exposure to extreme heat or cold
- Sudden loud noises
- Birth

Symptoms of Trauma

Typically, the following are the first symptoms to develop after an overwhelming event:

- *Hyperarousal:* This can include increased heart rate, difficulty breathing (rapid, shallow, panting, etc.), cold sweats, tingling, and muscular tension. Mentally it means an increase in thoughts, racing thoughts, and worry.

- *Constriction:* The nervous system focuses all its resources on the threat by constricting both body and perceptions. Blood vessels in the skin, extremities, and internal organs constrict to make more blood available for the muscles, which are tense in preparation for defensive action. Constriction alters breathing, muscle tone, and posture.

- *Dissociation:* This is a separation of awareness from physical reality, which protects from the impact of escalating arousal. Dissociation protects from pain and is a means of enduring what is beyond endurance.

- *Denial:* This is a form of dissociation requiring lower levels of energy. In this case, the disconnection is between the person and the memory of or feelings about a particular event (or series of events). There may be a denial that an event occurred or an assignment of unimportance to the event.

- *Feelings of helplessness, immobility, or freezing:* If hyperarousal is the nervous system's accelerator, immobility is its brake. When both of these states occur at the same time, a feeling of helplessness results. It is a feeling of being completely immobilized and powerless to act. The body feels paralyzed.

The following are other symptoms that tend to surface concurrently with, or shortly after, trauma (several of them can, however, show up later):

- Hyper vigilance

- Intrusive imagery or "flashbacks"

- Extreme sensitivity to light and sound

- Hyperactivity; restlessness

- Exaggerated emotional and startle reactions to noises, quick movements

- Nightmares and night terrors

- Abrupt mood swings (rage reactions, temper tantrums, shame)

- Difficulty sleeping

- Fear of going crazy

- Avoidance behaviors

- Attraction to dangerous situations
- Frequent anger or crying
- Abrupt mood swings
- Amnesia or forgetfulness
- Fear of dying or having a shortened life

The final group of symptoms includes those that generally take longer to develop. In most cases, they will have been preceded by some of the earlier symptoms (although there is not fixed rule when a symptom will appear).

- Excessive shyness
- Diminished emotional responses
- Inability to make commitments
- Chronic fatigue or very low energy
- Immune system and certain endocrine problems, such as thyroid dysfunction or psychosomatic illness, particularly headaches, neck and back problems, asthma, digestive distress, spastic colon, severe premenstrual symptoms, and eating disorders
- Depression, feelings of impending doom
- Feeling like the "living dead"—detached, alienated, and isolated
- Reduced ability to formulate plans and carry them through

The symptoms of trauma can be stable (ever-present) or unstable (come and go), or they may remain hidden for decades. They rarely occur individually but in clusters.

Biological Nature of Trauma

Responses to threat are primarily instinctive and biological and secondarily psychological and cognitive. There are three innate action plans: fight, flight, or freeze. The arousal cycle looks like this when a threat occurs:

1. Muscles tense; search for source.
2. Mobilize the body and mind; produce adrenaline and cortisol.

3a. Fight or flight (discharge energy). The nervous system is no longer aroused, returning to a state of equilibrium if the threat is handled.

or

3b. Freezing response (dissociation). This is an immobility response with the nervous system still highly aroused if the threat is not handled or is overwhelming. The integration cycle is incomplete and is not able to be completed in the immobilized state.

Physiological Processes During Trauma

The human brain is divided into three distinct layers, with each playing a part in a person's response to trauma.

* The reptilian brain (instinctive), called the brain stem, is the oldest part, evolutionarily speaking. It controls a person's basic functioning such as heart rate, breathing, and survival instincts.

* The limbic (emotional) mammalian midbrain, developed with the advent of mammals, has more refined responses to the environment, giving people feelings and emotional responses that allow for more nuanced interactions.

* The neocortex (rational) is the latest development in an evolutionary sense and allows even more complex manipulation of the environment, with symbols and representations that are increasingly complex.

Memory and Trauma

Our nervous system is designed to integrate stimuli from our environment and from our internal organs to mobilize the organism to approach or avoid situations for our survival and growth. Our nervous system has a storehouse of experiences called memories from which it draws to help assess the safety and desirability or danger and aversiveness of situations.

At around eighteen months the hippocampus starts its neurological function of integrating. Our *implicit* memories (that is, impressions of our raw sensations, pictures, and emotions) start to be integrated into what is called *explicit* memory, which is an awareness of this data as factual (i.e., "I know I am remembering this information about something") and as autobiographical (i.e., "I associate myself experiencing this historical event"). Our autobiographical experiencing can be either from an *observer* position outside of our bodies or as a *participant* through our bodies.

Later through these memories we create an autobiographical narrative or story about our life that helps integrate all our life experiences into a whole.

When you experience trauma, however, the hippocampus in the limbic system either is flooded with the stress hormones cortisol and adrenaline and stops its integrative functioning or is bypassed by dividing attention away from the hurtful stimuli to something more neutral (as in sexual assault when a victim leaves the body awareness and focuses on a picture on the wall). The hippocampus needs focused attention to integrate sensations, emotions, and pictures with facts and autobiographical memories to create a story that can lead to understanding, safety, and healing. (You will engage in focused attention exercises later to demonstrate this.)

Also when you experience trauma, neural pathways to the prefrontal neocortex, which assesses and orchestrates a plan of action to address challenges, are impeded, leaving primary attention to be focused on emergency reactions in the brainstem of fight or flight or the more extreme reaction of freeze. When appropriate action cannot be taken to return the body to safety, these emergency states become the common mode of functioning.

Daily life is filled with sensations, impressions, and emotions that do not get fully integrated to varying degrees and can lead to unconscious reactions in our lives. For example, I was scared as a child by our neighbor's large German Shepherd dog, who I was told was in the war and was vicious. I encountered him free of his tether rummaging in the bushes while I was coming home from ice skating one dark winter evening when I was about twelve years old. I at first froze but then slowly moved past him while clutching to my skates as a potential weapon. Ever since, even though I have had several dogs as pets, I have a wary reaction around German Shepherds, despite being told they are friendly. I am conscious of this event but still might have this reaction until I re-experience enough safety with this type of dog or the memories of the incident. Over the years I have become friendlier with dogs in general, and my current dog is my best animal friend.

Severely traumatized humans have a much harder time dealing with high stress or restimulating experiences, for example, when confronted with situations reminding them of past trauma. Their rational brain may become confused with the triggering of implicit memory stimuli, have a lack of explicit memory data, and be in conflict with instinctual responses. Under these conditions, the following happen:

- The nervous system remains in a state of arousal.

- Even if the threat is gone, the brain and the body react as it still exists and continue to put out the fight or flight chemicals.

- Excess energy becomes bound in the body and the mind.

Transforming trauma involves integrating instincts, emotions, and intellect such that they work together rather than against one another. The integration of the triune brain connects people to the source of their innate vitality. We are provided with the opportunity to realize our true full potential as human beings, realign with our spirit, and regain a sense of life purpose.

Animals without the more evolved brain mechanisms of humans deal with overwhelming threat also with fight, flight, or freeze responses but do not have the capacity to remember and prolong the trauma response in the same way that humans do.

The restimulated traumatized person is dealing with the overwhelming implicit-only memories and scrambling to make sense of their reactions that they cannot rationally explain. They feel hyperaroused physically and unvalidated emotionally or mentally in the absence of data that can make sense of their state. This can lead to all manner of compensatory behavior that looks "crazy" to others and even to themselves (e.g., hiding under their bed when hearing a dog bark, avoiding certain people that remind them of their abuser, or avoiding social contact altogether).

Approaches to Healing Trauma and Breathwork's Contribution

Clinicians and healers were dealing with healing trauma long before the neural functioning of the brain was understood. Extensive practice by sensitive and intelligent individuals over decades had already established a repertoire of approaches to working with trauma that are more effective than others. As always, what works for some does not work for others. Neurobiological research has filled in many gaps in our understanding and given us a sound basis on which to both test the results of different approaches and experiment with new discoveries.

Mind-Based and Hypnotic Approaches (CBT, Tapping, DBT, Hypnosis)

A traumatized nervous system is deregulated. Healing involves bringing a person's functioning—physically, mentally, and emotionally—back under their conscious regulation. Traditional psychotherapies have long recognized that trying to bring the physically traumatized system back to regulation with just cognitive tools is long, arduous, and most often frustrating for both the client and the clinician. Mind-body approaches were developed out of necessity because they take into account the mind-body synergy. Ideally they even bypass the artificial dualism of mind and body and work with the human as a whole functioning being. Nonetheless, trained as we are in the Western world, we still use our prevailing lexicon hoping not to miss the forest for the trees (i.e., using mental divisions to try to restore organic wholeness).

Dan Siegel, MD,[47] has led the way in applying neurobiological research to the Mindfulness approach to working with trauma. He helps clients assemble the chaotic stimuli of overwhelming life events into an integrated pattern and then link them into a coherent narrative that helps implicit-only memories be woven into an explicit autobiographical narrative that makes sense and helps them feel safe in their lives. In so doing, the individual also integrates the right hemisphere, which is the storehouse of strong emotional data, with the left hemisphere, which searches for a linear account to "make sense" of his or her life experiences. Mindfulness approaches can be combined with coherent breathing (five to six breaths per minute), which pairs a parasympathetic response to activating stimuli and supports this with cognitive reinforcement.

One of the most popular forms of psychotherapy in the Western world, Cognitive Behavioral Therapy (CBT), has conducted a number of research studies with healing trauma. CBT is primarily a mental approach that enlists clients to restructure their thinking to produce different behavioral results.

One such study concludes that CBT achieved as good results as medication therapy, and there is some indication that the combination of the two is a bit better than either in isolation. Still, this is around 20 percent recovery, which is only slightly better than no treatment at all (see Bessel van der Kolk, MD[48]).

Bessel van der Kolk, MD, director of the Mass Trauma Recovery Center, became impressed with a hypnosis variant in treating trauma because the results of various studies showed higher recovery rates of 40 to 50 percent. This technique involves putting the client in a mild hypnotic state while introducing a gradated reintroduction of the triggering stimuli. Freed from the most aversively triggering stimuli in their lives, those in the midrange of trauma symptoms were able to regulate themselves at a significantly higher level sustained over longer periods or indefinitely. They have also successfully employed *tapping,* in which a client learns to self-stimulate acupuncture meridian points and free energy flow while desensitizing the triggering stimuli. Both of these methods seem to go deeper into the client's subconscious control and again work better than just cognitive methods for restoring functionality for the midrange of traumatic symptoms. He also noted that trauma impacts differently depending on the developmental stage at which the person is at the time of occurrence.

A number of other creative therapeutic approaches are now combining mental and physical techniques, some of them involving a coherent type of slower breathing like Dialectical Behavioral Therapy.[49] I applaud all these efforts that bring neuroscience, clinical expertise, and human compassion together to address one of the most devastating problems we face as humans: overcoming the wounds of our past and ceasing to perpetuate them in the future.

Therapeutic Breathwork

Therapeutic Breathwork builds upon the advances of the previously mentioned forms of trauma treatment while adding another highly significant element not utilized in any other forms, the *activating breath*. In Therapeutic Breathwork clients are coached to engage in another way of breathing that mildly activates the limbic system (sympathetic nervous system) through increasing the breath volume in a safe setting. This allows formerly implicit-only or partially integrated stimuli to resurface and be more fully integrated with safe outcomes, as in my case with the German Shepherd. This is facilitated through the assistance of the "observer" breathworker and the "participant" client into an integrated story—often reinforced with the use of mental suggestion (affirmations or "inner child" visualizations that signal safety to the body, which will be introduced later in this chapter). This reprograms the chaotic emotional responses and negative story the mind reached (or was told) to explain the disjointed reactions to life experiences.

Since traumatic overwhelming stimuli can happen at any developmental stage in varying degrees, the negative stories are prime to be created in broad themes reflective of the developmental challenges of that stage (see the discussion of body themes in Chapter Five).

- *Prenatal/after birth:* "I'm not safe" (fragmentation)
- *Year 1:* "I am not enough or don't have enough" (abandonment/ deprivation)
- *Year 2:* "I'm not in control" (overpowering or seductive manipulation/ abuse)
- *Years 3 and 4:* "I can't express my feelings" (emotional suppression/ guilt and shame)
- *Years 4 and 5:* "I can't express my gender" (gender judgment/ confusion/alienation)
- *Years 5 and 6:* "I can't have fulfilling love" (intimacy block/betrayal)

Of course, traumas around these themes can happen or be reinforced at any period of a person's life. Healing involves relinking our emotions, sensations, and pictures with more resourceful outcomes than being frozen and self-talk that is continuously negative (e.g., "I am not lovable").

Therapeutic Breathwork precipitously engages the sympathetic nervous system to help reprogram what has been frozen in the fight-or-flight mechanism. As such, fears arise and are breathed through consciously and integrated. Energy thwarted by trauma and unavailable for more creative endeavors than being on continuous "red alert" or hypervigilant is thereby recovered. It does not anesthetize fears that might be appropriate for the person's well-being (e.g., wearing a seatbelt). But it helps put the original fears in a workable context to be understood and the energy of the fear to be integrated into more conscious use.

Pathways that had been cut off to the prefrontal cortex are now activated in resourceful ways, and clients "make sense" to themselves and can make productive choices based on present needs rather than operating in the trance state of past trauma.

Personal Account

Beverly, a healing practitioner with a PhD in nursing, had done a number of breathwork sessions dealing with the aftermath of incest and was participating in a breathwork practicum before she was triggered at home and did a spontaneous breathwork session with a caring friend (who later became her husband). She was able to integrate her frozen implicit-only sensations into a coherent, empowering autobiographical narrative.

"Near the end of my thirty days of self-rebirthing for the breathwork practicum, I experienced a spontaneous breathwork. Let me explain the breathwork and why I still look back on it as a significant experience.

"I am healing from physical and sexual violence perpetrated by my father during eleven years of my childhood (ages two to thirteen). Until two years ago I chose to forget this part of my childhood, leaving large gaps in my childhood memories. Forgetting is cited as a common survival mechanism in child abuse literature. A large part of the recovery and healing of these childhood memories has taken place for me since I began breathwork one-and-a-half years ago. I am thankful for the breathwork technique in my life. I believe this process has facilitated the healing and integration of my very traumatic childhood in a relatively short period of time and with great gentleness.

"A childhood memory or flashback (the term used in incest jargon) precipitated my breathwork. A special male friend was visiting me for the day. While sharing an intimate moment, he lay next to me, holding me. Just the way he held me triggered the flashback. Suddenly I was thirteen years old and the man holding me is my father. I felt that he was holding me and fondling my breasts. I felt the rage and terror of a thirteen-year-old child. She could not speak or scream or cry—she was immobilized.

continues

"At the same time I was aware of a voice inside me saying, 'Keep breathing,' and fortunately I did. I began Therapeutic Breathwork breathing. I was able to breathe and come back to the present to realize I am the thirty-five-year-old Bev: my body is my own, and the man who is with me I had invited and was choosing his touch and closeness. I breathed and took my little girl from my father. I protected her and took my power.

"During all this, I had bolted away from my friend, but he gently kept one hand on my back even though he had no notion of what was going on. His touch was an anchor for me to the present. I was in terror. Eventually, after what seemed like hours to me but was probably only minutes, the terror released with the breathing. I felt a release from the past. I had felt my inner child's anger, rage, hate, and shame and forgave her.

"I then was able to share with my friend what was happening for me—reminding myself to keep breathing while doing so. Fortunately I'd chosen to be with a compassionate man! He held me; I received his love and nurturing. I continued the Therapeutic Breathwork breathing. I felt so vulnerable. I went into the fetal position, and he cradled me against his chest. I feel like I suckled at his chest. My child felt nurtured and cherished. After another undeterminable time, the breathing cycle completed itself. I came back with a new awareness and acceptance of myself.

"I share this as my most significant breathwork for a few reasons. I feel the breathwork process became my own. To have spontaneously used the Therapeutic Breathwork breathing during a traumatic memory means I truly trusted the breathwork process. I listened to my inner voice and again trusted and responded to it. Knowing I have integrated this process helps me face the fear of more memories.

"Being able to breathe through this experience resulted in a healing and a learning for me, rather than staying stuck in the past. The insights and realizations gained during the breathwork are mine to keep and are very empowering. I can now choose to let go of my old beliefs that have been directing my being in my adult life.

"Finally my relationship deepened with my inner child. A common experience for survivors of incest is to feel 'crazy' when having flashbacks and thus discount the memory. Having stayed with my inner child during the flashbacks, then bringing her back to the present, affirmed this memory as a real part of my life—a part of my life I can now put to rest."

Other forms of breathwork that activate the parasympathetic nervous system (pranayama, coherent) are also useful in helping consciously regulate the traumatized nervous system but do not always address well-encapsulated (highly defended) areas of trauma. This can lead to well-controlled states of peace at the price of passion and full empowerment. The judicious use of both slower than normal and faster than normal breathing maximizes the chances of recovering full potential. The caution with Therapeutic Breathwork is the possibility of a flooding of the limbic system without resolution, which is tantamount to retraumatization. This is why training is required in its usage that is both technical and personal. The clearer the breathworker is concerning their own trauma that may have produced blind spots for them, the less likely they are to miss the signals of the client around their triggers. Fortunately, the course of trauma treatment is over a period of time that allows for adjustments and can be very forgiving, given the goodwill and commitment of practitioner and client. Even my miscalculations or blind spots have led to great healing when I have owned them and engaged in an honest dialogue that provided a new model of relationship healing for the client. For example, earlier in my career, having strongly encouraged a client to express anger before they were fully ready but then recognizing this, I was able to apologize and work through what could have been another overwhelming experience with an authority figure for the client. Healing came out of my "mistakes" (i.e., talking too loudly, being too animated, pressing my client to express, or myself expressing the feelings my client was afraid at that point to express) as long as I, the practitioner, was able to own them and work through them with the client. Again, when you are practicing this form of breathwork, you have to be aware, sensitive, and boundaried as well as operating within one's scope of practice in your respective profession (i.e., getting adequate training).

Foundational Concepts and Exercises for Healing Trauma Combined with Breathwork

This section summarizes the concepts and intervention techniques that have proven most effective (based on the research of Levine[46]) and are most amenable to be used in combination with breathwork in the treatment process.

RENEGOTIATING

Renegotiation is awakening the capacity for heroism and actively escaping the traps of trauma. It includes the following:

- Employing the elements of the original trauma (e.g., through memory, visualization, or spontaneous symptoms) combined with strengths and resources unavailable at the time of the event (e.g., imagining a protective figure intervening for them)

- Interweaving missing pieces (strengths, resources) with the incomplete defensive actions of the trauma, creating a new and complete experience (e.g., feeling an inner power that mobilizes defensive action through protective movements of the body and finding one's voice)

- Strengthening and building resistance to future trauma (seeing the self thwarting a future threat)

- Establishing a healthy aggression (an essential part of the recovery), which is the renegotiation from trauma to empowerment (acceptance of personal authority); in the immobility state, assertive, aggressive energies are inaccessible (e.g., initiating kicking with feet, hitting and/ or pushing away with hands, using a commanding vocalization, etc.)

Breathwork can use renegotiation in allowing for the unfreezing—the discharge and completion of the cycle of fight, flight, or freeze—by giving permission to deal differently with the sensations and feelings that empower the client. The process literally helps make new neural connections. It allows for the loosening, the softening, the going into and the coming out, back to the flow of life. The breathwork process then permits the reframing of limiting beliefs, in particular the experience and belief of helplessness through use of affirmations and making a coherent narrative of their life.

I will present some simple exercises that you can adapt during a breathwork session when working with traumatized clients or clients who you suspect may have been traumatized. Many of these exercises have been modeled from the work of Peter Levine, who has pioneered in the field of trauma recovery. It is suggested that you go through the exercises yourself as you read this chapter. If that is not practical, at least do them for yourself at another time before trying to lead a client through them.

Exercise

This first exercise helps you use the felt sense in the body, which is an awareness of one's sensations to help ground and feel safer.

Get in a comfortable position. Breathe easy and close your eyes (keep them open if it's more comfortable; it is important to give traumatized clients this option for their safety).

Wiggle your feet a bit and notice what you are feeling in your feet. Hot or cold? Are they comfortable or uncomfortable? Does one feel different than the other? Now feel your calves. What are you feeling in your calves? Hot or cold? Are they comfortable or uncomfortable? Does one feel different than the other? Now feel your thighs. What are you feeling in your thighs? Hot or cold? Are they comfortable or uncomfortable? Does one feel different than the other? Now feel your hips. What are you feeling in your hips? Hot or cold? Are they comfortable or uncomfortable? Does one feel different than the other? Now feel your stomach. What are you feeling in your stomach? Hot or cold? Is it comfortable or uncomfortable? Now feel your chest. What are you feeling in your chest? Hot or cold? Is it comfortable or uncomfortable? Now feel your neck. What are you feeling in your neck? Hot or cold? Is it comfortable or uncomfortable? Now feel your head. What are you feeling in your head? Hot or cold? Is it comfortable or uncomfortable? Now feel your body as a whole. What are you feeling in your body? Hot or cold? Is it comfortable or uncomfortable?

Notice what you observed about yourself in doing this exercise. Was it easy, uncomfortable, or annoying? Were some parts of your body easier to feel than others?

Simple body awareness is often foreign to people with trauma, and it may make them uncomfortable or confused because being in their body threatens that they will reexperience discomfort that seems to have no resolution. They may also shut down to the degree they feel nothing or outright refuse to do the exercise. Be understanding, compassionate, and patient. Being able to do this with safety could be a huge victory for someone living in fear of the pain stored inside them.

continues

Now close your eyes and choose a part of your body that stands out for you, either because it is uncomfortable, numb, or disconnected or maybe just because it occurs to you when asked. Focus for a moment on this area and imagine you can send your breath into that area like a stream of soothing energy surrounding and massaging it gently. If you cannot feel this, just imagine it is happening as best you can.

This is a more advanced body sensation exercise and may need some practice before people with trauma can do it. When they can, it is a major victory. It may take a while before they would attempt this on their own, but when they can, it is significant progress. These are all steps in becoming safe and taking active participation in self-healing.

Journaling the results of these experiences and reviewing them at a later time can be useful in deepening results. Note what you experienced in doing this—not only changes in sensations but also your emotions or thoughts associated with the sensations. Working with a safe partner can also be beneficial.

CREATING SPACE

This concept means creating space or room for new learning in the body and the mind, other than the fundamental fracture or split from the instinctual response of fight or flight.

Exercise

Get in a comfortable position. Breathe easy and close your eyes or keep them open if it's more comfortable. (It is important to give traumatized clients this option for their safety.) Breathe into your heart area and invite an image or a felt sense of someone you care about and who cares about you. See them smiling and opening their arms toward you; if this feels comfortable to you, imagine them giving you a hug. See whether you can relax and notice how much you can take in their care for you.

Again, you can briefly journal or share with a partner what you experienced in doing this.

This is a major step in creating space in a client's body and mind for what he or she chooses. It is not an attempt to cover up or deny negative feelings but, on the other hand, not to get stuck in the position of negative feelings being the only ones possible in his or her system. Again, it's a victory on the road to recovery. If the client cannot safely imagine such interaction, the exercise is not a failure. It is an accurate reading of their level of safety and important data in the treatment process. Acknowledging to the client that it is important that he or she is able to tell the truth about what is safe and what is not can be the positive outcome of this exercise.

RELEASING ENERGY

This technique means releasing the residual energy frozen in the body due to overwhelming threat and the override of the rational mind that inhibits the instinctual response

---

Exercise

Get in a comfortable position. Breathe easy and close your eyes (keep them open if it's more comfortable). Locate an area in your body that you sense holds traumatic memories. Ask that part of your body what feelings it is holding—fear, anger, sadness, all of them? Ask that part if it is willing to express and release these feelings. If so, listen to and feel this expression (if it helps, you might imagine yourself as a child expressing these feelings). Give permission and affirmation to that part of you and ask it to be a fully functioning member of your body and that it has permission to continue to express its feelings whenever it needs to. Notice what you discovered in doing this exercise.

This is an advanced and powerful exercise in your healing toolbox.

The more comfortable you are with doing these exercises yourself, the more effective they will be with your clients.

HELPING TO CHANGE ONE'S MIND

This technique includes helping to change one's mind, drawing a different conclusion other than one of helplessness or worthlessness.

Exercise

Briefly witness and recount an event in your life that is hurtful and/or frightening and unresolved—that is, one that still evokes uncomfortable feelings when recalled. Choose one that you feel you are ready to work with and will not be overwhelming for you.

Now review the event, seeing yourself giving protection to yourself and witnessing a more positive outcome for yourself. Without denying the negative aspects of the event, remind yourself what useful skills, conclusions, or insights about yourself or the world that you reached as a result of having revisited this event. See to what degree you can accept that both the negative aspects and useful conclusions can be held at the same time.

The ability to accept both negative and positive parts of the event breaks the sense of total entrapment and enables the individual to find their power in all life situations. If you cannot do this for yourself, you will have a difficult time helping your clients do it and probably will not be very convincing. Affirmations written in the energy psychology protocol use the format: "Even though I (state their negative reminder phrase, e.g., "am afraid of my abuser"), I deeply love and accept myself." The rewiring of the negative programming can be done only when the feelings associated with it are somewhat activated.[50] This is what happens in a breathwork session.

CHANGING THE COURSE OF INSTINCTUAL RESPONSE

This technique is developing the power to change the course of instinctual responses in a proactive way, role-playing a healthy response to the traumatizing stimuli with a client.

Exercise

This role-playing requires some degree of ego strength and willingness on the client's part. Let the client push against a pillow you are holding while their eyes are open and thinking of what it is they would like to push out of their life. Verbalize this clearly before beginning. Encourage simple but as strong and commanding a vocalization as possible (e.g., "Get out," "Get away," "Go away!"). Offer enough resistance to make the client really work but be successful in pushing you away. Keep eye contact and have them be in the present, not go into a trance of the past. Let them throw away the pillow at the conclusion and breathe fully and feel their power from head to foot. This can be done standing or lying down (more vulnerable).

This can be highly empowering and can be repeated over the course of treatment to mark growth and confidence. Go only as far as the client is willing and capable of sustaining strong expression. Avoid letting your feelings push them further than they are willing to stretch (as I learned earlier in my career) or you can overwhelm or even reinforce trauma in the client.

INCREASING BELIEF IN THE INNATE WISDOM OF THE BODY TO HEAL, TO RENEGOTIATE

Let the client suggest an empowering exercise (either protective or proactive receiving). Give a variety of suggestions if necessary (e.g., hitting, kicking, pushing, asking for contact, saying "no" or "go away," saying "I want you," saying an affirmation strongly, etc.) . Work in cocreating affirmations about the body's innate wisdom to heal and have the client cite examples of this truth from his or her life (e.g., "My body knows how to heal itself as I support it")—evidenced by my headache going away as I breath into it during a breathwork session.

Many of these exercises are also demonstrated and integrated into a Therapeutic Breathwork session in the videos cited in Chapter Five.

A Major Effect of the Trauma Is a Loss of Emotions as Signals

Chronic physiological arousal and the resulting failure to regulate autonomic reactions to internal or external stimuli affect people's capacity to utilize emotional signals.

The psychological function of emotions is to alert people to pay attention to what is happening so that they can take adaptive action.

People who suffer from post-traumatic stress disorder (PTSD) no longer use arousal as a cue to pay attention to incoming information. Instead, they tend to go immediately from stimulus to response without first being able to figure out the meaning of what is going on; they respond with unmitigated fight-or-flight reactions. When unsuccessful at eliminating threat, it causes them to freeze or, alternatively, to overact and intimidate others in response to minor provocations. Thus, the abused can become "abusive" in an attempt to be safe.

After having been chronically aroused, without being able to do much to change this level of arousal, people with PTSD may (correctly) experience just having feelings as being dangerous. Because of their difficulties using emotions to help them think through situations and come up with adaptive solutions, *emotions merely become reminders of their inability to affect the outcome of their life and therefore are assiduously avoided.*

Another Major Result of Trauma Can Be Loss of Self-Regulation

The lack of development, or loss, of self-regulatory processes in abused children leads to the following problems with self-definition:

- Disturbances of the sense of self, such as a sense of separateness, loss of autobiographical memories, and disturbances of body image
- Poorly modulated affect and impulse control, including aggression against self and others
- Insecurity in relationships, such as distrust, suspiciousness, lack of intimacy, and isolation
- The combination of chronic dissociation, physical problems for which no medical cause can be found, and lack of adequate self-regulatory

processes is likely to have profound effects on personality development. These may include the following:

- Disturbances of the sense of self, such as sense of separateness
- Disturbances of body image; a view of self as helpless, damaged, and ineffective
- Difficulties with trust, intimacy, and self-assertion

Personal Account

Jessica, a nurse, recounts a traumatic childhood event that had profound implications for her self-esteem and trust in social and intimate relationships. She was courageously able to work through them with the aid of Therapeutic Breathwork and to be more resourceful in her current life challenges.

"During this breathwork session with Jim's help I remembered the source of my pain. I was able to return to me being a twelve-year-old and to reexperience what had happened to me then and how those events paralleled my current state of feeling betrayed. My past event was that I had just been sent home to northern Minnesota by my sister, whom I had lived with for almost two years. I had been told by her I was more of a bother than a help to her. I had not been able to meet her expectations of caring for her children. When I arrived in Minnesota, I was encouraged to make the choice to go to a foster home rather than return to my parents. I agreed to a foster home; upon meeting my foster parents, I soon realized it was a mistake.

"They could not let me in their hearts; they were still enmeshed with their last foster daughter, and after realizing I was so unlike her and as they tried to instill in me how she was, I closed up my heart to them. I concentrated on doing what I had to in order to live there but put my energies into being a good student. In the spring of that year I realized how lonely I was and attempted to start making some friends. It was not too long before I was approached by a group of very popular girls asking me to join their group. In order to join their group I had to prove I was brave, which meant skipping school and hitchhiking into a nearby city for a day. I had good grades and attendance and felt I could go along with this adventure.

continues

"Soon the day came, and I went with one other girl, who was the leader of the group. All went well until we actually arrived in the city. Around lunch time, a car with boys pulled up and started talking to us. The girl I was with seemed to know the boys, and when they asked us to go for a ride with them, she agreed. I felt scared, as this was something I had never done before, and I questioned her but in the end agreed. The ride ended in a park. There I was gang-raped by three of the boys; she was not. After the rape she told me all the bad things that would happen to me if I told anyone. Somehow I managed to get back to my foster home. I kept my vow of secrecy and also refused to be friends with the group, using any excuse I could think of, and continued to excel in my studies. My anger was directed at myself for believing I could have girlfriends and then being used and at the boys who hurt me, but most of all at myself for not making good decisions. I felt what happened to me was my own fault because I didn't check out the things they did and just believed their stories of how much fun they had in the city. I felt I had no one I could trust and that I truly wasn't cared for by anyone.

"Through Jim's gentle guidance and with my breath and commitment to healing, I began to understand I had never forgiven myself for this sad event. Because of my embarrassment, and feeling unworthy, I did not tell my truth to the girl or to people who might have helped me. I took it upon myself to try to decide what was best for me. Because of my age and position, my world view was pretty limited, and my adults may have given me help, if I had allowed myself to ask.

"This situation was much the same with losing my job (currently) and taking it on myself to solve my problem without asking for help. This time I was stopped in my tracks with a fix. I believe it happened to give me time to come to my senses and to use all my resources rather than to try to do everything on my own.

"In this breathwork I got the initial essence of what was going on. As the days and weeks went on I revisited both the past area of my life and my current situation. I continued to work on forgiveness for myself and to put the pieces together. I learned at the deepest level the importance of telling my truth and to love the courage of my little twelve-year-old. I began to understand more clearly my strength and how I can use this example always in my life. This truly was one of my most important breathwork sessions. I have deep gratitude.

continues

"This breath session began a journey that continues to weave in many directions. As I told myself my truth, I was able to see the areas of my sexuality that need healing. I took the six-month course on survivors of sexual abuse and continue healing this area. I began to find ways to do truth-telling checks on myself and to start trusting others with my truth. I began to discover how fragile my sense of safety is and how to create safety with my truth. I also began to truly empower myself with breathwork. This was a mighty session."

Breathwork provides the venue in which to explore and detach one's sensations and emotions that may become heightened from the stories and judgments about them.

This may happen spontaneously, or the breathworker may play a helpful role in having the feelings become associated to different outcomes.

The following are more advanced techniques in healing trauma.

TRACKING

Tracking is being mindful of the body sensations and images, allowing the individual to become conscious of previously hidden instinctual responses by doing the following:

- Tuning into the inner landscape

- Joining with the animal instinct within that is central to renegotiating the trauma response

- Following the mystery of the internal landscape—-specifically, following body sensations (hot, cold, loose, tight, numb, frozen), images, feelings/emotions, thoughts/beliefs

- Always changing—even if frozen or numb with the belief "nothing will change," it will change simply in contacting it

The breathworker notices or asks about parts of the body that may become charged or cut off during the increased breathing. The sensations or feelings are then focused on or "breathed into" to help move stagnant energy and make it more available for healthy expenditure.

Exercise

Locate a chronic or typical sensation somewhere in your body. Close your eyes and breathe into the feeling. Describe the feeling in physical terms (hot, cold, loose, tight, numb, frozen, size, shape, color, movement); then in images (looks like a ball, sword, lightning bolt, etc.); then in feelings/emotions (mad, sad, glad, scared); then in thoughts/beliefs—messages from and about the sensations ("let go," "be kind to yourself," "own your strength"); and finally in memories or imagination—"When might your little one have experienced these kinds of feelings when they were young?" Now notice any changes in the sensation. What other sensations or areas of the body seem connected to this sensation, and do they help strengthen or dissipate the sensation?

You may start with relatively benign sensations with your client and work up to sensations in highly traumatized areas of the body.

APPLIED IMAGERY

The following are ways to use guided visualizations either scripted or spontaneously created:

- Image-based solutions use the right hemisphere of the brain for perception, sensation, emotion, and movement rather than the left side's standard cognitive functions of thinking, analyzing, verbalizing, and synthesizing.

- Trauma produces changes in the brain that impede a person's ability to think about the event and actually accentuates the capacity for imaging and emotional sensory experiencing around it.

- The part of the brain that creates cognition and language takes a hit from the biochemistry of the trauma experience.

- The imagistic, emotional, metaphoric, and sensory avenues of the right brain are sensitized, hyperactive, and over-functioning.

- Trauma needs an oblique route through the imaginal realm, using metaphor and symbolic language to help manage the symptoms, find a sense of safety, recontact to the "most whole" self, and make language a viable avenue again.

- Guided imagery is a benign form of focused, strategic dissociation—a consciously deployed dissociation with a purpose. The client deploys the trance state in a conscious positive way (fire with fire).

- The healing content of imagery meets the ugly matter of trauma exactly where it lives—in the world of the right brain's reverie, sensory, fragments, and feeling.

Traumatic memories are not absorbed by the thinking brain the way ordinary memories are. They are shelved in disconnected sensory fragments, somatic sensations, and muscular impulses in the more primitive areas of the brain and are walled off, disconnected from awareness and inaccessible to cognition (implicit-only memory).

Trauma goes underground until there is internal readiness to let it surface and an external precipitant to bring it forth (see Naparstek, Belleruth[51]).

Ironically, it may not be until a person has established enough safety in their life that their organism is prepared to deal with the overwhelming trauma, say, ten, twenty, thirty, forty, or fifty or more years later. Healing does not happen on a linear time schedule.

Exercise

This exercise is useful for contacting your feelings or emotional body that may be walled off from awareness or too scary or painful to access directly.

Arrange your body in a comfortable position, sitting or lying down. Breathe up your back on your inhale and down your back on the exhale, forming a circle of breath and intention around your body, affirming nurturance and safety in this sacred circle. Breathe into your heart and ask for an image, picture, or felt sense of yourself as a little one. Take whatever comes. (I, like about one-third of folks, do not see pictures right away, so you may have to go with just an inner sense of your little one. When with

continues

a client, ask what their child is feeling and what the child wants most with the client right now.) Ask your child what he or she is feeling and wants most with you right now. Listen with your heart and accept whatever sense you have. Thank your little one for connecting with you and let them know that who they are, what they feel, and what they need and want is a very vital part of you. If it OK for you to use these words, say to your little one, "I do not want to live without your innocence, curiosity, and loving openness to life. I know that I cannot immediately make everything better in our life, but I can promise you this: I will not leave you. You are precious to me, and I want you back fully in my life. I want to learn and grow together." Notice how your little one reacts to this invitation. If they are cautious or even unbelieving, that is OK. It is honest. You have to start establishing trust with them, which may take time. You can deepen your trust with your little one by letting them take the lead in some things until they get that you are not just out to manipulate them and make promises about a partnership you don't keep. They probably have had to take a backseat to many things in your life. If it is OK with you, ask your little one to take your hand and show you their safe place. It is important that you do not prescribe what it should be, but just feel their little hand in yours and see where they bring you if they are ready to do so. They may not be ready until you have built up more trust together. You have to learn to trust that their feelings will not overwhelm you. If they do bring you somewhere, know that this place is sacred to them and that it is a privilege to have them show it to you. When you have their permission, you may have a part in decorating their safe place with the favorite things you share together. Ask, if you are willing, that they meet you there regularly—every day if you are both willing. Again, do not make any promises you are not willing to keep. This can be a place of rejuvenation of your spirit. Also, this can be an important haven to which to return if and when they show you their scary, sad, or angry places in which they need your support. Breathe together for a moment, making contact with your little one, and express gratitude for their renewed pres-ence in your life. Then with a few deep and clearing breaths, come back to your adult awareness, but continue to hold the space for your little one in your heart.

This is a door opener with which it is vital that you follow up and make the imagery of inner feelings your own—perhaps a little ritual you do every morning before getting out of bed. I do it while I am bathing. Make it fun or neither of you will want to show up. Ask your little one each day what they feel and what they need or want. Then listen with your heart. If you are connecting with your emotional body, the answers will be simple and fairly direct. It does not mean you can do everything they ask, like taking the day off from work. But you can perhaps offer to do something special after work. Make it a real relationship. No, this will not make you schizophrenic. The little one is of course a metaphor for your emotional body, but it's a useful one that you can use until you are in sync with all your past and present feelings. Again, play with it, be creative, and make it yours. When you do this, you will be in a much more authentic place to share the tool with your clients.

You may find it useful to journal responses to "What I learned about myself in doing this exercise is …" and "How I could use it with my clients or others is …"

I often ask my clients to create their own meeting with their little one and ask them three questions:

- Where are you little (childhood name for themselves)?
- What do you feel?"
- What do you need and want?

I ask my clients, when they are able, to journal their little one's responses and bring the responses with them to sessions. Sharing these can be instructive in the healing work.

PENDULATING

This involves establishing a natural rhythm that guides back and forth between the past (unresolved) defeat and the present (resourced) experience, allowing for the formation of a new experience. Specifically, this utilizes the following:

- Positive feelings and/or sensations and distressful feelings and/or sensations

- Tracking regions, like a flashlight—shifting/moving between polarities of expansion/contraction
- Following the rhythm of exchange and flow

Exercise

Close eyes or focus on something in the room. Make contact with your inner child. Ask them to take your hand and lead you to their safe place. Let them know that you will help keep this place safe for them. Ask your child if for the purpose of healing they are willing to show you to a scary place for them with your protecting companionship and agreement to return to a safe place whenever they want. When in the scary place, let them know they are now protected and resourceful and that they no longer need to live in fear of this place having power over them.

If clients are willing and able, shuttle back and forth two to three times between safe and scary places. Have clients do it on their own and report results to you.

Movement gives clients a different sense of who they are, not trapped in either safe or unsafe place or in their feelings. They come to know a full range of human experience.

A rule of thumb I have as a practitioner is to always experience an exercise for myself before leading clients through them.

The breathworker, having helped a client find their safe place, can then assist the client to explore scary memories and/or feelings, always reinforcing the option to return in his or her imagination to the safe place whenever he or she wants. This becomes an invaluable tool for life outside the session, which has been linked to both the client's breathing and thinking. When ready, the client can lead himself or herself through this exercise. This is a great victory in self-recovery.

RESOURCING

This includes finding instinctive resources for successful self-defense when overwhelmed in the original event. These resources can become available and useful with the tracking process for bringing current strengths, insights, and support along.

- These resources help resuscitate positive feelings and sensation. A resource could be a person, animal, nature, a guide, a safe place, a person, and maybe even the breathworker (with care around boundaries, transference, and projections). These external resources help unlock internal resources such as self-talk and affirmation, courage, and faith.

- The human nervous system is wired for expansion and pleasure, not constriction and holding. The limbic brain has more fibers for pleasure and exploration than for pain and protection. Explore with the client and find the resources that speak to him or her.

- The breathworker's skill is in listening to the client's story as well as the story the body is telling (e.g., frozen legs, feet jittery, jaw clenched, breathing restricted) and then suggesting resources that fit their story and help redirect it.

- I often suggest that my breathwork clients bring a resource of their choosing with them during a session (e.g., inner child, spiritual figure, animal guide, ancestor, deceased grandparent, parent, partner, friend, element of nature, etc.).

- I suggest breathworkers experiment with inviting a resource with them on their breathwork journeys before recommending this to clients.

GROUNDING AND CENTERING

This includes reconnecting the individual directly with resources naturally available in the body. Grounding can involve literal physical grounding exercises for getting into one's legs, feet, and floor of the pelvis (e.g., dance,

Qi Gong, *T'ai Chi*, Bioenergetics). The exercise "Increasing Strength and Resilience," below can also serve for grounding.

Centering can involve slow breathing, visualizations of serenity, comfort and support.

- Trauma disconnects people from their bodies, and the sensation function has been impaired.

- Grounding and centering reconnects a person directly with resources naturally available in the body.

- Grounding and centering allows a client to come safely into contact with the body.

- Trauma dissociates. Love sweeps us off our feet, but trauma pulls our legs out from under us.

- Survival energy left unresolved in the body needs to be grounded and connected to the earth.

INCREASING STRENGTH AND RESILIENCE

Grounding and centering also reconnects a person to a sense of strength and resiliency. With this, the individual is poised for successful defensive reaction. Useful experiences here are those that help the client bend without breaking and bounce back.

Exercise

Play lively music. Move and sway to the rhythm. Start to bounce up and down. Feel your feet connecting to the earth. Let your legs bend and straighten. If physically capable, come off the ground and bounce back like a cat. Feel the power and strength in your legs. Sense the resilience in your legs and your whole body. Come back to resting position and feel the strength and resilience still there.

With trauma people either stiffen and brace against it or collapse. They can't easily spring back. The physical experience of being able to "spring back" can be renewing.

DAILY ORIENTATION AND COMPLETION

After a person emerges from immobility, help will be needed to reorient the individual to a world that often appears quite different from before. A highly important element in long-term recovery is to help clients stabilize their progress and self-empower with daily self-care practices (e.g., journaling, exercise, prayer/meditation, connecting with nature, etc.).

This may also involve helping clients to do the following:

- Completing cycles and finishing tasks, especially involving self-care, which can include everything from paying the rent to joining the gym. Completing the cycle discharges the energy that had been fueling the symptoms of trauma.

- Establishing equilibrium, such as by improving self-soothing talk and using calming breath.

- Always orientating, including reminding the client to be in the here and now and noticing sensations, colors, and smells.

- Noticing where there is enjoyment or hyper-vigilance.

- Restoring self-regulation.

- Moving in different levels of arousal, with a range of regulation and a full range of responses other than 25 mph to 90 mph.

- Increasing freedom from worry.

- Sorting out beliefs that were reinforced with frozen fear.

- Regulating perception accurately, not seeing everything as representative of trauma.

It is not possible or necessary to hold all of these thirteen methods of approach and techniques in the forefront of your awareness when dealing with the healing of your clients. Yet periodic review of this toolbox can be valuable when dealing with stuck places in the therapeutic process.

Personal Account

Christine, a social worker and breathworker, did her own recovery work with the aid of Therapeutic Breathwork and is now able to help others with disabilities including a severely abused infant she has adopted.

"I think about how I was in my life before breathwork and realize that I was fearful of everything and everyone. I didn't know that I was afraid of my own anger but thought it was always someone else's that I feared. I would actually avoid places and people so as not to have a confrontation on any level. Now I welcome confrontation and see it more as a conversation of passion and opinions and learn so much about myself and the other person. I am not paralyzed in fear anymore and feel the world is big enough for everyone's opinion, so I don't avoid anything or anyone anymore. The plus about discovering these concepts is that I am able to breathe through any situation now without becoming invisible or small. I was taught the technique, so I was able to work on my process alone and utilize a facilitator when I wanted. I was trained in the technique later to facilitate others and realized that my benefits of breathwork continue and multiply. It develops a level of consciousness in me that keeps me clear and focused for being the best support to another. The daily practice of breathwork is so integrated and automatic that I am almost clearing blocks constantly. Every situation is an opportunity to be conscious. It offers some people a chance to actively move, clear, and be without having to have a physical voice."

Spirituality and Trauma Healing

To pray is to breathe, and the possibilities of prayer are for the self what oxygen is for breathing.

—SØREN KIERKEGAARD, *SICKNESS UNTO DEATH*

Without a sense of purpose or meaning, trauma often remains at best an unfortunate circumstance of which one is left to make the most. Being able to put the traumatic events into a larger context can help bring completion that rational explanations fail to reach.

For many, dealing with trauma is greatly aided by including the spiritual dimension directly in their healing process. I would go so far as to say that unless clients can find some sense of purposefulness in overtly tragic life events, healing may never come to completion and leave subtle elements of debilitating fear and/or resentment around their fate. They may not have a model of spirituality or even have antagonistic responses to spiritual concepts or language because of negative religious associations. It does not take overt talk about spirituality to include purposeful dimension in the healing process, a personal meaning that fits for them in their life. In supporting this, you can observe resources in an individual that go beyond reason or will power, emotions, or behaviors. Call these resources what you will, they can be crucial in relieving much suffering on the healing journey. If not summoned through prayer or meditation, they may be invoked with "inner child" visualization, guided imagery, or just love of family. This has been research verified again and again.[52] Bessel van der Kolk stresses the concept of helping the client "reinstate the instinct of purpose" when working with trauma. This does not require imposing your value system but helping clients recover their own sense of purpose in life.

It behooves you as the practitioner to explore and utilize the resources of the client rather than to impose or try to replace the client's spiritual approaches with your own. Even in the case of religious trauma or avowed atheism, there is often a way that individuals relate to higher principles of kindness, respect, and compassion, for example, that go beyond their egocentric interests and point to a higher aspect of themselves.

For those open to it, after validating their basic organic self-preservation instincts of anger and self-defense, they may be ready to accept a resiliency in their spirit. This can put the trauma in a larger context than just a victimization that leaves them permanently damaged or something they think they deserved for wrong doing or unworthiness on their part.

When enough safety has been established, clients may begin the forgiveness process, which always starts with forgiving themselves for being involved in the trauma. As counterintuitive as this may sound, our child emotional system often harbors self-blame for any hurt. Here is where it is critical to distinguish blame from responsibility. Blame attributes causation and recrimination or deservingness of punishment for any pain or hurt in one's life. Responsibility gives one the power to deal with their responses to their life experiences, helping them be "able to respond" in more resourceful ways. For example, if I accept blame, I am stuck taking ownership of everyone's part in the creation of the experiences and the imputed punishment if these experiences do not please everyone. If I deny responsibility or blame others for my condition, I am left in a powerless victim position with little recourse but to carry the scars around. Responsibility gives me the impetus to find new resources and take a proactive role in not only my healing but also my thriving as a result.

Forgiveness is a key to re-owning my healing and thriving power. Step 1 in the forgiveness process is to forgive myself by first giving up allegiance to the belief in permanent damage. Yes, it is true a lost limb may not grow back after a car accident. But that does not mean that I am "essentially" less of a person deserving love and respect than before. The second part of step 1 is that even though there may have been tragic loss (e.g., the death of a child), there is some learning or gift in the process that I can claim (e.g., a restoring of faith in the kindness of those who share my pain or a sensitivity to the suffering of others, that I may own that I did not have before). This in no way whitewashes the tragedy or removes all grief, but it does leave me more resourceful and empowered. Beyond what the individual may learn from their involvement in the traumatic circumstances, there can also be a learning from all parties involved; the community or context around the occurrence can also benefit from the healing taking place. The individual, the relationships, and the world can become more conscious through the healing. Having a good start on step 1, I then more easily may go on to the further steps of forgiveness: 2) forgiving the others involved, 3) accepting that part of the other that forgives me (though in their personality they may continue to hold a grudge), 4) giving up claim to punishment of the other or myself, and 5) restoring harmony in my relationship. The last step does not mean necessarily becoming friends with the other who might engage in abusive behaviors. It could mean establishing strong appropriate boundaries, while not seeing the other as having power over me or vice versa.

The spiritual perspective can help give a broader meaning to the trauma and consequently further catalyze the healing process.

In the beginning of many breathwork sessions, I ask clients if there is someone whose spirit or presence they would like to have with them on the breathing journey. This could be anything from a traditional religious figure from childhood to a grandparent or pet. I accept what they suggest and have seen that it has been a great comfort to many. It also reinforces their ability to invoke spiritual assistance on their own in life. At times I will suggest their "inner child" or someone they have told me is important to them if they are at a loss to mention anyone.

If their physical or emotional body starts to get overwhelmed with the increased volume of breathing during a session and they begin to "check out," I will ask them to invite their "little boy" or "little girl" into their heart. Since about one-third of people do not visualize well, I make sure to say to bring an image *or* felt sense of their child into their heart. If we have not in our work already established a safe place for that child, it is always the first order of business to have them imagine their child taking their hand and leading them to the child's safe place, if they are ready to do so. Encouraging the client to continue to breathe while engaging in this visualization not only keeps them awake but also helps them get into a receptive place to have their feelings. It's often more permissible to empathize with their child's feelings than to directly own them as an adult at first. Once the safe place has been established, the child can be used as a "consultant" in future work either in sessions or on the client's own. This process directly relates to the success of the "pendulating" work with trauma (i.e., having a safe place to which to retreat when too much scary emotional material surfaces).

With clients open to it, I will further explore making their spiritual guidance part of their breathing homework. It can deepen their personal relationship with spirit immeasurably. Even if the client is not open in their personality to using spiritual concepts, this does not prevent the practitioner from addressing their spirit and the "Great Spirit of Life" silently to partner with them in bringing the highest good to the client in their healing and to give help in knowing how best to serve the client (prayer). I recommend this practice before every session. The growth of the practitioner's spiritual awareness and clinical skills is one of the greatest rewards I know for being a breathworker. The medium for spirit is highly enriched in breathwork. It is more than coincidence that in a number of languages the word for *spirit* and *breath* are the same. I consider it truly sacred work guided by spirit (the principle of life) and that my greatest service is most often to get my personality out of the way and to let this spirit of aliveness work through me. Amazing healings happen when I do, both for my clients and for me.

Basic Treatment Principles in a Breathwork Healing Trauma Session

"No matter how strange things get, know that with every breath, you are becoming that which you have always been."

—ERIC MICHA'EL LEVENTHAL

Many of these principles apply to any healing work, but I find them especially important when working with a client experiencing the symptoms of severe trauma. The principles stem from my clinical work going back to 1970.

SAFETY FIRST

Establishing basic safety starts even before treatment officially begins. Clarity in working agreements and safe boundaries are often issues violated in the client's original trauma and easily restimulated if the practitioner is unaware in their initial contact, be it on the phone, by email, or in person. Being open and accepting on the one hand and clear and boundaried on the other are the parameters of safety that lay the groundwork for a successful partnership in healing.

Practitioner boundaries involve knowing what service can be provided and what cannot. The former category includes coaching in the art of breathwork, informative feedback from the healing approaches in which one is trained, support in the therapeutic work during the contracted time of sessions and what availability is offered in between sessions, cost and payment options for the service, and general expectations for the length and outcome of the service. What cannot be provided are guarantees of outcome, the expectation of unlimited availability, techniques outside the scope of one's training, and the implicit promise of meeting all the client's needs. Practitioners who deal with trauma and use techniques involving nonordinary states of consciousness such as breathwork need to have done enough of their own personal work to be aware of their own needs and how to not get them confused with the needs of the client (see *The Ethics of Caring* by Kylea Taylor[10]). Unless the practitioner has enough inner safety with their own dynamics, it will be nearly impossible to convey safety to a traumatized client.

COLLABORATIVE APPROACH

The truth is no practitioner knows all of what is best for a client. If the practitioner does not listen to and learn from the client, the practitioner is operating from general theory rather than interaction with a live person. Establishing a collaborative approach from the onset takes the practitioner out of the role of the expert who knows the answers and is responsible for the healing. Clients must know they are the experts on themselves and ultimately responsible for their own healing as they are helped to marshal the resources around and within them and have the courage to stay with the process. The practitioner has some tools to share, but how or if they are employed will depend on the feedback, willingness, and readiness of the client. All of this requires a working rapport between the two. The practitioner cannot impute, demand, or legislate trust. That will only come when the client experiences the genuine openness of the practitioner to learn from them and work collaboratively.

The following are practitioner qualities that can be honed to help this process:

- *Warmth:* A genuine empathy and acceptance toward the client
- *Clarity:* An ability to stay focused and clear on the process undertaken and the tools used
- *Enthusiasm:* A vitality and attraction to one's work and desire to meet the client's goals
- *Empowerment:* Directing the process toward the client's growing sense of self-confidence and expertise in self-care

EXPERIMENTAL ATTITUDE

Given a working rapport, the practitioner must be flexible enough to abandon a technique that is not working rather than abandon the client. This is easier when practitioners do not expect themselves to know all the answers and have established a collaborative approach. I always suggest "homework" that clients agree to try, letting them know that making changes in their lives is more important than just what goes on in our sessions. If, however, a suggested journaling or visualization is not implemented outside of our sessions, I assume it was for a good reason. Perhaps it was too soon or too threatening to write vulnerable entries about themselves at home. Our job is to move past it and find what does work. Even during sessions I will ask a client if he or she willing to experiment with a way of breathing, moving, or vocalizing. First, the agreement gets them on board with it. Second, it reduces some of the performance anxiety around having to do it right—"It's just an experiment to see what happens," not a device to make something happen. Regardless of the outcome, we learn from it. For example, if I hold a pillow and have the client look at me and push on the pillow and say, "Get away," I let him or her know as an experiment I will not take it personally. Then if the client feels angry, sad, scared, empowered, or nothing, we learn from it. Seeing that I really mean this usually not only gives the client permission to do more experimenting with new behaviors and ways to deal with challenges while in session, but also in his or her life.

FORGIVENESS

The more these principles are established, the easier it becomes to deal with the inevitable issues and challenges that arise in the emotionally charged setting of trauma work. Sometimes I can get animated in a session and perhaps raise the volume of my voice, a trigger for my client. I will notice the client's discomfort and ask them about it. If clients have the courage to admit their discomfort and I have the courage to admit my lapse in awareness around their trigger and the willingness to apologize for it, we may accomplish more in that interaction by way of healing life patterns (e.g., relationships with authority) than years of theory and analysis. We begin to accept our so-called mistakes as learning opportunities that actually create more safe closeness and self-forgiveness. As practitioners, we cannot legislate safety. By accepting that at times we may inadvertently re-create circumstances of discomfort or threat but that these are invitations to work through old woundings, we may provide invaluable opportunities for our clients. This may not happen immediately and in some cases may even give them the opportunity to set a boundary and leave treatment. It is here the practitioner's forgiveness of themselves and their clients is most tested and can be a life-altering release.

SELF-CARE: VICARIOUS TRAUMA, COMPASSION FATIGUE

This is what happens when a practitioner's boundaries are compromised and he or she begins to take on their client's issues. Breathwork encourages practitioners as a point of ethics to continue their self-healing work, rec-ognize the signs of their own distress, know when to take a break and/or seek appropriate support and revitalization, and maintain healthy peer and supervisory relationships. All of the principles and techniques mentioned here in the service of assisting others in their healing process apply to our self-healing. Owning your own needs is important if engaged in helping others with theirs. Finding a trusted helper and committing to your own process has been recounted by so many of the counselors' and healers' sto-ries in this book. I hope they will inspire you to do likewise.

The next chapter will help you discriminate among the life and body themes that clients present when coming for counseling, breathwork, and other healing modalities. These themes can give you important clues as to what healing paths they are on and how you may best serve them, while employing the strengths of your own themes in the process.

Chapter 5

Therapeutic Breathwork and Body Themes: An Integrative Approach and Neuroscience Hypotheses to Six Major Breathing Patterns

"Breath conquers thinking, because one must 'let go' when breathing out. The power of breath goes beyond the judging mind …. Whenever we exhale, the air we breathe out is compassion. It is the breath of giving or releasing. Inhalation is receiving. Like birth and death. Inhalation is a constant birth. In this way, we say, we are able to receive life."

—JAKUSHO KWONG, *Zen in America*

This chapter introduces body-theme classification, including its structural, behavioral, and proposed neurological correlates. In addition, I demonstrate how an integrative approach can be used in Therapeutic Breathwork and other healing modalities most effectively with these body theme patterns for both clients and practitioners.

A *body theme* is an enduring constellation of structural and characterological positions a person takes toward their life that reflect basic beliefs about themselves and their world and how to survive and grow in it.

Each stage of human development is associated with a body theme that is adaptive in its formation but can become dysfunctional in its persistence into adult life. All humans face the basic themes of safety, abundance, control, freedom of expression, sexual identity, and intimacy, and they adopt attitudes and postures around them. Each body theme operates on a continuum from fear based and restrictive to integrated and highly functional. The theme of safety in the first stage of life, for example, may be portrayed in one's body as fragmented and highly constricted or as secure, sensitive, and integrated. All humans pass through each of the six developmental stages and have elements of each body theme. For most humans, however, one stage will stand out with regard to its structural and characterological influence. The defenses of this stage will most often serve as the default mechanism when the person is under stress later in life. This is useful for a practitioner attempting to help a client under duress in both assessing and successfully addressing the client's core issues with techniques that access and help integrate both sides of the brain.

Therapeutic Breathwork has evolved as an art and science since the late 1970s and is used directly and as an adjunct in a wide variety of healing professions. Breath awareness and breathing techniques have been used for thousands of years for health and human growth. Therapeutic Breathwork's faster than normal breathing focuses on newly evolved techniques that help release cognitive and emotional blockages to healthy and optimal functioning often related to trauma and developmental dysfunction, as you saw in previous chapters. As such, Therapeutic Breathwork and similar dyadic forms of breathwork differ from yogic and coherent breathing techniques that activate the parasympathetic nervous system and help induce a regulated state of calm and relaxation. Those types are what are called *maintenance breathing*, which I recommend for daily well-being and health maintenance. Therapeutic Breathwork also employs a more active breathing rhythm and activates the sympathetic nervous system to address holding patterns in the emotional body and the physical body. The principal technique involves a dyadic interaction in which a practitioner helps guide a client through a thirty- to sixty-minute breathing session. A connected breathing rhythm induces a mild altered state of consciousness that can produce heightened awareness, make unconscious material more accessible, and facilitate more resourceful cognitive and emotional connections. The facilitator's role is to assist clients to embody more functional coping and evolving in the face of the experiences that have compromised their healthful functioning. Beyond this, the goal is to help them find the gift or treasure that often lies beneath their "wounding" and unlocks doors to their full potential. This takes place through teaching a more full and free breathing, providing a safe atmosphere for clients to explore and experience more cognitive, emotional, and spiritual integration, and assisting them to translate these states into more satisfying and purpose-filled lifestyles.

Neurophysiology of Body Themes

Desmond Tutu once remarked that in the African language the word *ubuntu* means a person becomes a person *only* through other people, underscoring the importance of social and emotional embeddedness to a developing child. Dan Siegel states that the importance of the first years may be that the brain structures that mediate social and emotional functioning begin to develop during this time in a manner that appears to be dependent upon interpersonal experience.[53] Eisenberg refers to "the social construction of the human brain" and argues that the cerebral cortex is sculpted by input from the social environment.[54] Stern proposed the "self" as developing within a series of overlapping and interdependent stages during the first years of life. Each domain of self-experience begins at a certain age but continues to play an important role throughout the life span.[55] Neuropsychobiological literature supports the idea of the maturation of the infant's brain as experience-dependent and embedded in the attachment relationship. The polyvagal theory posits three phylogenetic stages of neural development in the autonomic nervous system and three corresponding levels of emotive and interactive behaviors cued by environmental/caretaker stress ranging from a myelinated parasympathetic (social engagement) to spinal sympathetic (fight/flight) to unmyelinated parasympathetic (freeze).[56] Yet, the "how much" aspect undertaken and debated within the nature-nurture question in recent research stops short of the psychological and somatic response that lies at its nexus since the mind/brain is contained within the body. This mind-body connection was first put forth by Reich's Vegetotherapy and later expanded upon by Lowen's Bioenergetic Analysis. In it, Lowen points toward "the etymology of emotion refers to movement, and muscles are the organs of movement. What happens mentally through characteristic ways of experiencing life affects physical expression."[57]

Bioenergetic Roots of Body Themes

Lowen's Bioenergetic Analysis typology of character structure depicts six basic personality foundations thought to exist on a continuum, with one character structure expressing more dominantly over the course of ensuing developmental stages. Attunement dysregulation between the infant/child and primary caregiver triggers a somatic adaptive response culminating in held muscular tensions during the critical developmental stages, from the prenatal period through early childhood. According to Lowen, each stage is characterized by a developmental need that must be met and integrated for the child to successfully thrive. Should a basic developmental need not be satisfactorily met, a fixation dynamically expressed as *character structure* is reflected in the body through specific muscular tensions/holding and breathing patterns. These holding/breathing patterns are unconscious expressions, reflecting the child's genetic endowment and the way in which the child responds physically to needs being met or thwarted by caregivers. For Lowen, the implicit model of health is an unarmored body structure that exhibits the openness and flexibility to deal with life with minimal need for any rigid defensive structures.

Other authors have since expanded upon Lowen's original typology, some adding subcategories and emphasizing different modalities of treatment.[58] What follows are the six character structures that I have developed based on Lowen's work:

- Psychic Sensitive
- Empathetic Nurturer
- Inspirational Leader
- Steadfast Supporter
- Gender Balanced
- Energetic Grounded

The neuroscience hypotheses behind the six developmental patterns presented in this book are meant to be suggestive of possible structures and functionality that are in the process of being validated through research. They offer possibilities for investigation based on current data.

Description of Body Themes and Breathwork Goals

The following sections describe the six body themes. The *Breathwork and Body Theme Training Video* that I created includes interactive exercises tailored to each of the six body theme's breathing patterns. The videos demonstrate the strong emotional releases and integration that can happen in combining bioenergetic exercises with connected breathing techniques and are an integral part of Therapeutic Breathwork training and certification. See the video at www.transformationsusa.com/lifelong-learning.php.

Theme 1: Psychic Sensitive— Safety vs. Danger in the Body and the World

The approximate age of emergence of the Psychic Sensitive structure is from prenatal to nine months. When this period is highly stressful, a pattern can develop in the body exemplified as "holding together" against fear of annihilation. The formative dynamic is thought to correlate with the primary caregiver's responsive style of ambivalence, hatred, or anger, supporting the formation of a negative core belief that the world is unsafe—a cold and hostile place such that the infant is cut off from experiencing the love of others. Again, it is the infant's response to the environment rather than specific behaviors the infant does or does not encounter.

Neurologically, at around six weeks, the infant is capable of interactive facial and eye expressions, making mutual gaze interactions possible. The already active amygdala, part of the limbic system,[59] gives the infant the capacity of having emotional experiences linked to outer events. Although the amygdala is best known for its function in *aversive* conditioning, this ability only matures sometime after birth. This maturation difference permits early attachment regardless of parental behavior. Until the capacity for aversive learning has matured, the infant will continue to turn toward an insufficient or abusive caretaker but will respond with stress and fear while doing so.

Bentzen[60] summarizes the responses of the three vagal branches of the autonomic nervous system when she states the following:

"The myelinated, social vagal system is active under conditions of normal inter-action, for instance when the baby smiles, gurgles and makes different noises to invite food, sleep or play. When the child is stressed, this organization gives way to the phylogenetically earlier fight-flight system. In the infant, this first means crying, and increased startle and gripping reflexes. With more intense activation, the infant screams while flailing and twisting in an increasingly disorganized manner. Finally, if there are no outlets for fight or flight responses, the most primitive system and the dissociative parasympathetic coping strategy become dominant. The infant withdraws, becomes passive and quiet or immobile, and shows little or no interest in contact or food.

"The prenate and neonate infant is beginning to develop a sense of separate self, and is mostly dependent on his caretaker for basic modulation of arousal. If frequently abandoned or treated with hostility, habituation to a constant level of fear and distress becomes the 'normal' resting state. This is thought to be the most common formative dynamic of this character pattern. Isolation impacts the emerging self-regulation, and if the infants' experience is not offset, the later formation of internalized objects of self and others will be hostile and depersonalized."

The ensuing basic right in question is, "Do I have the right to exist?" (Do I exist? How do I exist in a dangerous world? Am I real?)

Figure 6 shows a diagram of the limbic system and prefrontal cortex. The limbic system is a rapid-scanning quick-response system that mediates the fight/flight mechanisms. The amygdala, in particular, has been shown to mediate fear responses. It is predominant in infancy before the cortical system and its higher cognitive functions have developed. Without inhibitory input from the prefrontal areas, over-activity of this system in infancy can lead to habituated fear based body and behavior responses later in life.

The infant's original feeling state is one of terror and rage at being cut off from parental love, which becomes deeply repressed as the body is experienced as an uncomfortable, unsafe place to be. The infant therefore tends toward fragmentation in movement with corresponding shallow breath. The major muscular tension is in the joints, with split energetics at the diaphragm and in mind-body; the tension exemplifies dissociation or disembodiment, disjointed and frozen with minimal breathing, and unfocused and operating in a survival manner with weak ego strength. The eyes generally appear distant, fearful, fixed, and vacant. The reaction to stress is to split off or dissociate.

Under these conditions, the growing child becomes increasingly more comfortable existing in the realms of imagination and speculation. The developmental challenge becomes one of existence versus need, with safety being the predominant issue and concern. Their unconscious theme is, "I can exist if I don't get too close (to my feelings or others)." Since they exist in their mind, for safety, a corresponding tendency is toward superiority to others with an air of "being above it all." In the most extreme, these individuals have a pattern of not being able to persist with undertakings or relationships long enough to be of lasting benefit. Figure 7 shows the body structure of a woman with the Psychic Sensitive theme.

Figure 6.

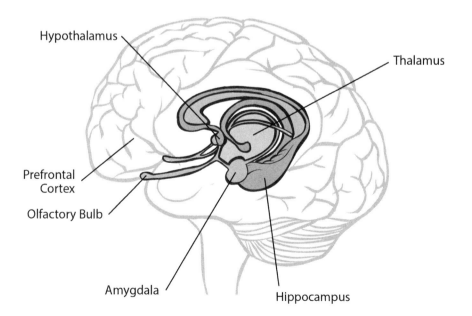

Figure 7.

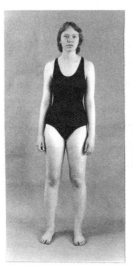 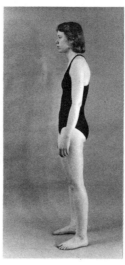

Psychic Sensitive Type

Face:	mask-like
Forehead:	flat
Eyes:	blank
Chest:	frozen; expanded
Abdomen:	contracted
Ankle:	frozen
Feet:	everted; cold
Skin:	undercharged

The fear-based polarity of the Psychic Sensitive posture is characterized by deep holding patterns in the core of the body and a habituated parasympathetic dissociative activation, which leaves the skin and the extremities cold. Movements are often stiff and clumsy, and there is little spontaneous movement. Breathing is shallow, and the general physical impression is of a person who has withdrawn as far as possible from aliveness. Bentzen cites Reich as noting primary blocking around the eyes and in the suboccipital-orienting muscles of the neck. The body is characterized by deep, "frozen" holding patterns in and around the joints, twists, and significant differences of organization between the right and left sides, as well as between different parts of the body. This somatic pattern has elements of the disorganized flailing of the infant in severe sympathetic distress frozen in a matrix of dissociated primitive parasympathetic inhibition.

Brennan typifies the correlates as hyperactive and ungrounded, with weak joints, and exhibiting energy blocks/loss at the base of the skull. Physically she notes a twisting of the spine; weak, thin wrists, ankles, and calves; and the head being held to one side. The defense pattern is one of withdrawal and disembodiment with a tendency to minimize self-expression and emotional contact, appearing distant, aloof, overly analytical, and logical.

Emotionally, the unintegrated Psychic Sensitive pattern personifies the lack of a sense of self. Associated with a history of splits between parental word and emotional (face/eyes) expression, anxiety and panic underlie estrangement from self and dissociation from inner feelings and the body.[61] There is deep fear and a lack of joy. Adults with the fear-based polarity of the Psychic Sensitive traits describe their inner experience of the self as alien, disconnected, fragmented, and deadened. The person is primarily identified with the mind and often distrusts and dislikes the body and its unruly feelings. The social world and other people are felt to be alien, stressful, or innately hostile. Therefore, there is a tendency toward difficulty in forming relationships and to react—rather than act—and move out into the world.

In its integrated state, the Psychic Sensitive is aligned with the underlying truth of their sensitivity and safety, bringing their free spirit into creative expression in the material, and with the ability to express safely in a balanced and grounded body. Most authors agree that the strengths of the integrated Psychic Sensitive state are sensitivity, psychic/intuitive abilities, and responsiveness. Other positive attributes include creativity and many talents, a rich inner world shaped by analysis, and intuition with a mystical connection. Integrated Psychic Sensitive abilities have contributed enormously to our culture via artists, visionaries, mathematicians, and creative endeavors in every field. As mentioned, each of us has some of that capacity to tap into and from which to benefit.

Personal Account

Pol, an accountant and sound healing practitioner, has strong Psychic Sensitive qualities. He has developed his artistic and creative sides into an integrated lifestyle that brings these qualities into practical and rewarding service.

"I have been combining breathwork with the use of live instruments and chanting through training from shamanic practices and sound healing programs. The results have been quite profound, and the experience is quite organic, meaning easily adaptable to what the client is experiencing."

BREATHWORK GOALS—PSYCHIC SENSITIVE

The life goals for this pattern are to fully arrive and to be present and alive in the world. Therapeutic Breathwork goals for this pattern are to increase awareness in the head and in the felt sense of the body through the breath and grounding techniques. This is done by emphasizing the following: increasing the inhale, mobilizing the chest to increase breath formerly reduced or cut off by fear, increasing tolerance and safety in experiencing life in the physical environment over time, and ultimately releasing rage and fear while gaining comfort and safety in the body. Encouraging too much breath too fast will produce a "leaving the body" response and perhaps a discontinuing of the work. It is important to build a sense of safety gradually in expanding the capacity to breathe and feel. When working with this theme, the practitioner needs to be well grounded to provide a safe, secure foundation for the client. Trustworthiness in words and actions, patience, and a willingness to commit to the work over the long haul are important traits in working with the Psychic Sensitive themes. Further, it is important to maintain steady and regular contact using genuine warmth and acceptance, to avoid double messages in communication, and to engage clients in the practice of daily applications of body awareness. Affirmations can be used to counteract fear-based mental programming. Physical activity should be stressed, and integrating safe touch can be helpful to reconnect with the body.

As a breathworker with a Psychic Sensitive structure, it is wise to be mindful of a tendency, when noticing a lack of response from the client, to withdraw and move further into your own head, engaging in an unconscious power struggle in an attempt to convince the client you are right; to lose touch with the client while under the illusion that you are better; or to try to save people with your "specialness and pure mind," all while avoiding feelings—especially negative aggression—yet getting affirmed on the ego level what was denied on the body level. Your goal as the breathworker is to give up any head game and let the process take place, allowing for short-term resolutions. Your strength as a breathworker is your sensitivity to others, your heightened intuition and spiritual connectedness, and your creativity.

Theme 2: Empathetic Nurturer— Abundance vs. Deprivation and Abandonment

The approximate age of emergence of the Empathetic Nurturer structure is the first year of life, exemplifying, when unintegrated, a pattern in the body as one of "holding on" against loss and deprivation. The formative dynamic is thought to be lack of early interpersonal nourishment and support or, less commonly, deprivation of physical nourishment. The environmental caregiving is seen as unavailable or weak, depressed, ill, or resentful of the differentiating needs of the child.

Neurologically this period is characterized by explosive neuron growth intimately shaped by the specific life conditions and interactions in the infant's new social environment. The primitive brain-stem structures are already functioning, and the mammalian vagal system will mature during the first several weeks.

The orbitofrontal cortex undergoes rapid maturation from birth to around eighteen months and is central to the ability to form attachments and relate in meaningful sequences.[62] This part of the brain handles emotional evaluation, which is positioned between the limbic system and the frontal cortex; emotional evaluation is central to the capacity for self-regulation of effect and the regulation of the autonomic nervous system, while also forming the basis of cognitive assessments.

The inner state of care-taking strongly activates the fronto-limbic cortex in the caretaker. In the infant, the orbitofrontal cortex is strongly involved in the internalization of love and safe caring. In addition, "being with" via identification coupled with imitation become linked together and form a "norm"—imitating more of the caretaker's treatment toward the infant and thereby losing self-agency, positive effect, and motor competency if the caretaker's presence is lacking .

Figure 8 shows areas of the frontal cortex involved in planning, logical reasoning, and appropriate social/emotional responses. As these develop, they modulate the raw emotional reactions of the limbic system to produce more appropriate responses to environmental stimuli. For example, if a child experiences chronic neglect, deprivation, or abandonment, the limbic system repeatedly reacts with a fight/flight or eventually a freeze (collapse)

response. Reasoning that the parents are there to provide for and protect them would inhibit this anticipated fear/collapse response. If the child
repeatedly experiences neglect, however, these neural and neurochemical
connections of "love and safe care" do not develop appropriately.

Figure 8.

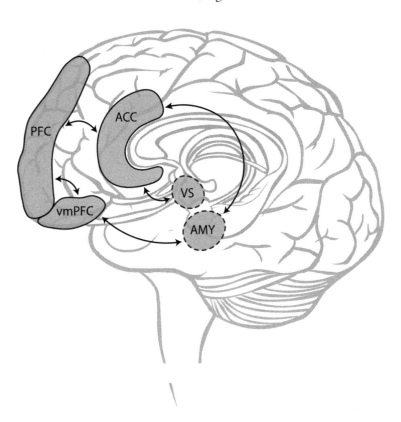

The basic right in question is, "Do I have the right to have?" (Is there
enough?) While the infant may have experienced some loving acceptance
by the mother, there is a corresponding feeling that what was given was not
enough, provoking the developmental challenge "need versus independence."
The correspondence and flow between the outside (environment) and the
inside (infant) set the tone for all future exchanges: abundance or deprivation.
Therefore, a central theme of anxiety develops around the issues of support
and nourishment and the fear of "not enough" love, food, care, and so on.

Since the right to be secure as a birthright has not been established, the body is underdeveloped and weak. Brennan postulates hypo-activity in a depleted energy field, which appears calm and quiet. Energy is held in the head, and the body has flaccid, smooth muscles; a cold and depressed chest; and a corresponding shallow breath. Totten equates this pattern as having tension in the jaw, held back in anger, with a desire to bite and attendant constriction in the throat. They also note energy being held high in the body with somatic energy constantly rising up, seeking the original nourishment not satisfied when younger. This correlates with a shallow inhale, a collapsed chest, the pelvis held forward, and the knees locked. The eyes are pleading and puppy-dog-like. The reaction to stress is collapse. Figure 9 shows the body structure of a woman with the Empathetic Nurturer theme.

Figure 9.

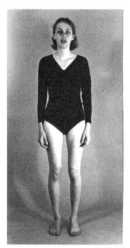 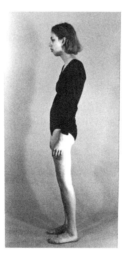

Empathetic Nurturing Type

Face:	lips full
Head:	inflated; tension at base of skull; jaw and mouth tension; scapula tension
Chest:	collapsed; sternum depressed
Back:	weak lumbar; longitudinal muscles clenched
Legs:	locked; thin
Feet:	everted; long and thin or flabby; body often tall and thin; weak and undercharged
Skin:	bruised easily

Emotionally, the fear-based polarity of the Empathetic Nurturer is most frequently associated with depression and a fear of abandonment and dependency. Inner rage over feeling abandoned is coupled with a denial of having any needs; therefore, the individual responds as either overly self-reliant or excessively needy. Deep-seated feelings of loneliness and the fear of being alone are met with disappointment and helplessness. There is a tendency to feel misunderstood. The lifelong strategy is a constant search for the place, person, event, and situation that will meet their needs, reliving fears about inability to survive alone. Therefore, the central theme is one of need and support, characterized in relationships of reciprocity with strings. The defense pattern is verbal denial and oral sucking.

Strengths and core qualities include the ability to be empathetic, to be serene, and to love directly from the heart. They can be a person of high intelligence and articulate with a sensitivity to injustice. In the integrated state, individuals with a predominate Empathetic Nurturing theme present as light, approachable, and warm with a yielding and receptive manner. Empathetic and compassionate with self and others and confident in their inner source, they have the ability to be happy and feel abundant with what they have. They are good in helping professions, do not over-identify with others, and are able to care for themselves.

Personal Account

Mari Lynn, an occupational therapist, has developed her Empathetic Nurturer skills for self-healing and professional service. She shares how she used breathwork to deal with her themes of loss and abandonment at a critical time in her life.

"Breathwork really helped me process the caregiving tasks and then the death of my father, which for me was the most profound experience of grief I ever had. I had a most difficult time with his death, and my Breathwork sessions were ultimately what lovingly helped me get through it. I highly recommend this for any type of grief work."

BREATHWORK GOALS—EMPATHETIC NURTURER

The goals for this pattern are to confront the fear of being alone, own the inner self as the true source, trust in the abundance of the universe, and learn to give with boundaries. Therapeutic Breathworker goals include the following: to support sustained charge without "doing for" your client; to bring up the breath into the chest gradually to a full inhale; to increase self-support, acknowledgment, and self-confidence; to increase awareness of, followed by, a decrease in the abandonment and depletion themes that can be assisted through use of affirmations; to increase energy in the legs and lower body, inducing a felt sense of strength and support; and to decrease the need to talk as an avoidance. As with the Psychic Sensitive theme, a gradual buildup of breathing capacity is important such that it can be sustained over time without collapse. When working with this structure, avoid "doing for" your client or becoming too important. Nor should you minimize, abandon, or deny the justice of their complaints. Project warmth, support, patience, and confidence in clients' abilities to help themselves, without promoting an inflated or deflated sense of self.

As a breathworker with an Empathetic Nurturer structure, be mindful of the potential toward several tendencies: feeding others and giving others what you originally wanted; colluding with the client through pleasing each other, culminating in the support of tandem stuckness and the client's increased confusion or the need to leave the helping relationship; needing the client to improve in order to feel you are enough and to get love; undermining the client's anger and aggression resulting in increasing client depression; and falling into the "Messiah role" while trying to be a better parent than the client originally had. Your goals as a breathworker include the following: contracting with clients that your role is to take care of them and their role is to take care of themselves; realizing clients have other goals than pleasing you; knowing yourself well before you "lay on hands" and become very important to clients; and communicating your feelings without setting up clients to take care of you through validation of your perceptions. Assign your client "healthy pleasures" and develop sensate intelligence. Inner child and boundary work are highly useful. Suggest movement therapy. Your strengths as a breathworker include your empathy, warmth, and understanding; your ability to verbalize your feelings; and your capacity to nurture others.

Theme 3: Inspirational Leader— Harmony vs. Overpowering or Seduction

The approximate age of emergence of the Inspirational Leader structure is the first to third years of life; when unintegrated it exemplifies the pattern of "holding up" against the fear of vulnerability. The basic right in question is, "Do I have the right to be free?" (from the manipulative needs of others).

Toward the end of the first year, many new cortical developments occur. From eight to fifteen months, the brain undergoes a massive pruning of synaptic connections in which unused connective possibilities are culled. Such pruning occurs several times during childhood and is probably related to qualitative leaps in effective and cognitive organization. At around nine months, the infant becomes able to manage much higher levels of pleasure and excitement, particularly in intense dyadic contact with the mother. From ten to thirteen-and-a-half months, a strong heightening of positive effect and lowering of negative effect is observed.

Neurologically, this elation reflects the development of dopamine circuits from the limbic system into the orbitofrontal cortex, which "comes online." The orbitofrontal cortex is central to the linking of externally experienced events with internal states and feelings. The right lobe, primarily related to emotional processing, is larger and has much stronger connections into the limbic system than the left one. This right-brain maturation allows the toddler to form an inner schema of the different emotional expressions of the mother, linking their inner sensory and emotional response. At the same time, the infant begins to have a sense of time, or temporal coherency, allowing formation of an experience-based representation and expectancy of future events, which are used to guide actions. In other words, the orbitofrontal cortex is the center of object constancy. However, the maturation of complete inner schemata seems to depend on the development of high levels of dopamine excitement in the relationship, and it may be disturbed both by insufficient arousal and by hyperarousal. Burton and Levy suggest that with insufficient arousal toddlers' representations remain more primitive and piecemeal. Hyperarousal, on the other hand, is thought to lead to unmodulated rage responses. Unstable interactions during this time can lead to dysregulation of these systems, disturbing self-confidence in a child's ability to relate to the environment in healthy ways. If the inner schemas become associated with continual power struggles, self-confidence may be contingent upon seeking high arousal and being in control.

Figure 10 shows the increasing influence of fronto-cortical systems on emotional regulation as the child continues to mature. Reward systems become more sophisticated and are mediated by cognitive functioning to a greater degree. Overpowering and/or seductive interactions, however, can lead to faulty reasoning and impaired cognitive schema, resulting in a mismatch between reasoning/planning and appetitive rewards. This mismatch can result in chronic affective hyper or hypo arousal, as well as deficits in the child's confidence for getting its needs met in a harmonious manner. Often the child tries to compensate for this mismatch by attempting to over-control situations that seem chaotic and unstable.

Figure 10.

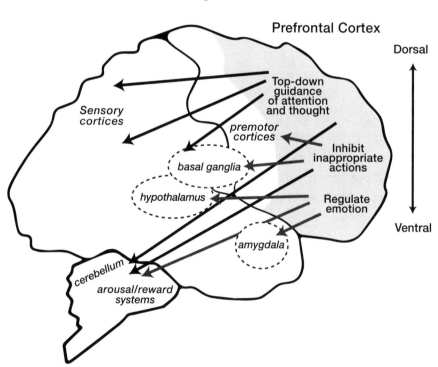

Having experienced oneself as being loved in a resource-secure environment, the infant feels confident enough to move with expansive curiosity into the environment. Utilizing increased independence via newfound physical mobility and in the exertion of will, the infant may be perceived as too threatening by parental egos, which may then respond with seductive manipulation rather than overt control. The child soon learns to play the game of power, predicated on the emotional premise that to expose one's feelings directly is to court vulnerability to seduction. What ensues is a struggle between the emerging independence/will of the infant and ultimate parental control of rewards, especially those of direct physical contact.

Bentzen states the two formative dynamics as embedded in the relationship to the mother. One theory is "mother as manipulator," in other words, one who induces the child to believe in the ability to manage by himself or herself, denying the infant's helplessness, or who is afraid of it and ignores any neediness and weakness, focusing only on strengths. In this stage of basic reality testing and subsequent modification of inner schematas, the mother does not help to test reality, so the infant maintains grandiose and unrealistic images of self and abilities. Another theory is that the mother is both over-excited by the accomplishments and over-identified with the infant. Rather than being with a containing, sharing, and regulating mother, the child is met with an escalating excitement that overwhelms, causing the child to lose track of internal feelings and activity in the surge of maternal affect and contact. The child then begins to avoid contact with the over-stimulating mother and, in the absence of regulating contact, forms a more partial schema of inner states and emotions. Driven by the inner dopamine high, the child dives into the sympathetic excitement and intense task absorption of the practicing child and denies the vegetative needs that would lead the child back to the mother about whom the child is now ambivalent.

The somatic holding pattern of the Inspirational Leader structure includes the following: tense legs, a tight pelvis, a tendency to walk on the toes, and a lifting of the whole body up by the shoulders. The gaze is magnetic and the manner engaging. The child may be described as having energy displaced upward and tends toward motor and verbal activity.

The practicing child walks on the forefoot. Falling reflexes in the arms and shoulders are just beginning to become active, and the arms and shoulders are used to keep balance as well as to handle objects and play with people. The child is "up" in its own body and fascinated with getting up on high things—climbing stairs, chairs, kitchen counters, or even refrigerators, often to the horror of parents and caretakers. The social charisma, excitement, and varied "language babble" are also typical of the practicing stage. The developmental challenge is "independence versus closeness" in relationships. The basic belief is that to give in to feeling is weak, and the corresponding reaction to stress is the need to control, rise above, and/or seduce.

Two subtypes characterize this pattern: the over-powering and the seductive. The over-powering type strives to win directly by subjugation of any opposition to its will, though manipulation may be used initially. The physical presentation suggests an inverted triangle with a muscle-bound upper body, with head and shoulders disproportionately large and waist/hips narrower. Legs tend toward the spindly. The gaze is compelling and powerful with eyes watchful and distrusting. Feelings are denied even to the self, and the infant must be ever vigilant and controlling for fear of falling down and being victimized by the parent again. This fear becomes predominant in the psyche and elicits violent defensive responses when triggered.

Figure 11 shows the body structure of a man with the over-powering Inspirational Leader theme: a muscle-bound upper body with compelling eyes.

Figure 11.

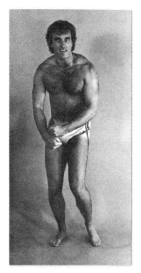 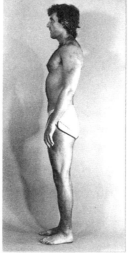

Inspirational Leader Type—Overpowering

Upper body: disproportionately large
Eyes: powerful and compelling
Base of skull: marked tension
Shoulders: large and rigid
Pelvis: rigid; undercharged; held in
Legs: oral (locked, thin)

The second pattern is more charismatic and seductive, using charm and wit to gain control. The body type is more evenly proportioned with smooth features and perhaps flabby, rather than strongly defined muscles and a hyper-flexible back. Beneath the surface is a solid layer of tension and fear, which is resistant to closeness much less penetration. The head-body split is more pronounced with this structure.

Figure 12 shows the body structure of a man with the seductive Inspirational Leader theme; even proportions with ingratiating expression and mannerisms.

Figure 12.

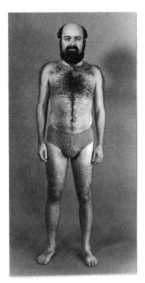 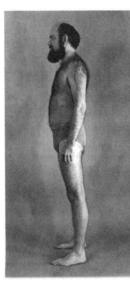

Inspirational Leader Type–Seductive

Face:	soft; innocent; intriguing
Back:	tight
Pelvis:	highly charged but dissociated, jerky quality
Body:	even proportions

Both types display an easygoing social façade, leading to immediate likability although of a superficial nature, since self-disclosure may be unlikely within relationships. The head is held high, with an active pelvis and blocked middle. Brennan states that head energy is hyperactive and then collapsing with energy and armoring in the chest/heart area, which is congested and split off.

Emotionally, these individuals find it hard to experience the self just as they are and are uncertain about whether they can have their needs met in a straightforward manner. There is a difficulty in showing vulnerability, for fear of being denied, being deeply wounded in the heart area. Verbal denial and explosions of controlled, balanced rage are the defensive pattern and reflect a more traditional view of narcissism.

In its integrated state, these individuals possess leadership qualities that help the individual rise above the situation and take charge without losing touch emotionally, with themselves, or those they lead/serve. They are strong, attractive, and energetic, exuding confidence with an ability to act skillfully in emergencies. They are able to let down and admit their vulnerability when appropriate as well as accept the support of others. Being in touch with their feelings is owned as a strength rather than a liability. They can seek positions of leadership in the world without needing to dominate but lead from their heart. These qualities are valuable in the world of commerce and politics and, indeed, in all service-oriented professions.

Personal Account

Sandra, an art therapist, has integrated her Inspirational Leadership talents into her work with some very challenging populations.

"At a summer camp for severely emotionally disabled youth, I facilitated circular breathing (a slower than normal Therapeutic Breathwork breathing technique) at the beginning of our Art Therapy sessions each day. Thirty teenagers surprised me by actually closing their eyes and doing the circular breathing without any disruption and without anyone refusing to do it, and they followed the directions perfectly as the room became totally silent. They were absorbed in the process. The camp director took pictures. She was amazed. It was later reported to me how it helped some of them during challenging situations in the following week, when, by themselves, they paused and did the circular breathing to bring their energy back to calm alertness.

"When facilitating healing for alcohol and other drug-addiction groups for a Native American social services organization, I taught circular breathing. A young male group member told me he was on the Huber Law detention program, working during the day and then returning to jail around 5 p.m. His wife had not brought his children to the jail to see him in over six weeks, even though he begged her to do so, over and over. One night he was writhing in his bed, in so much pain, missing his children. Then he remembered to breathe as he had been taught to soothe himself and soon fell asleep. The next day, the children were there to visit him."

BREATHWORK GOALS—INSPIRATIONAL LEADER

The goal for this pattern is to incorporate the underlying truth of the safety in interdependence and the awareness that mutually supportive and harmonious relationships are possible. Therapeutic Breathwork goals include the following: to increase safety in loss of holding up a type of control through power games (e.g., being "one up," having the last word, etc.); to complete the exhale fully to relax and let others closer to their heart; to increase awareness, safety, and pleasure of body feeling and sensations, while decreasing "great ideas" as a substitute for feeling; to increase strength and safety in legs, reducing fear of falling; and to increase safety in surrender with others. Journaling and automatic writing may be given as homework to augment healing outside of sessions. Trustworthiness, strength, and patience should be communicated. It is imperative that the breathworker not project the need to control the client. Instead, the goal is to work with the client, minimizing expectation or demand. Don't buy into the "mask" presented by the client of being in charge. When working with Inspirational Leader structure, approach from a partnering perspective rather than engaging in a power struggle.

As a breathworker with an Inspirational Leader structure, be mindful of a tendency toward your internal illusion that you need no one to help you, which is the unconscious control-power game and which sets up the winner/loser dynamic culminating in a lack of therapeutic "looseness." Your goal as a breathworker is to center yourself and work from your heart-space, not solely from your head or will, while communicating in honest, appropriate self-disclosure with your clients. Your strength as a breathworker is your ability to hold the vision, to motivate and inspire your clients while giving rise to their own strength, and to overcome adversity.

Theme 4: Steadfast Supporter— Freedom of Expression vs. Humiliation

The approximate age of emergence of the Steadfast Supporter structure is from the second to fourth years of life; when unintegrated it exemplifies the pattern of "holding in" against the fear of humiliation and shame. The basic right in question is, "Do I have the right to act?"

The earlier general state of pleasurable dopamine excitement is now followed by a period of anxious, depressed, shame-responsive hypothalamic-pituitary-adrenocortical (HPA) activity, starting between twelve and fourteen months. This phase heralds the beginnings of the development of social inhibitory capacities in the child. Great importance is placed on the development of shame. This intense swing from a positive sympathetic to a stress-deflated parasympathetic state is thought to activate further development of the frontolimbic structure (affect regulation) and the maturation of the orbitofrontal cortex (object constancy and emotional assessment). The fearfulness, depression, sensitivity, and separation anxiety described at this stage of child development fits the descriptions of the emerging adrenocortical function. This affective state is triggered by normal misregulations as well as shaming interactions.

The toddler is abruptly plunged from a state of pleasurable, high-dopamine sympathetic excitement into a sudden stress-filled parasympathetic vagal activation. The child's excitement is sharply inhibited, the heart rate abruptly slows, body and limbs lose tonus, the head hangs, and the face loses tone and blushes. The legs may even give way. The child feels lost, and the mother seems like an alien being. It is now vital that the mother can regulate the infant out of this state of intense shame, since the toddler's immature nervous system does not yet know how. The child will probably try to make contact with the mother to reestablish the lost regulatory flow and, with it, the good inner feelings. If all goes well, the mother will connect and stay in contact with the toddler until "back on their feet" again. Through this kind of interaction, the toddler's sense of object-constancy deepens as the child incorporates conflict and painful dystonic feelings, as well as healing, in representations of "being with." Around eighteen to twenty-four months, signal shame is becoming an internal guiding system that is strengthened in toddlerhood as the child becomes increasingly sensitive to the signs of disapproval.

Figure 13 represents shame as encoded not only at conscious levels but also at deeper preverbal levels where it manifests in body postures and breathing patterns. This deep sense of shame is often difficult to access through rational thought but can be addressed directly by working with the breath and body.

Figure 13.

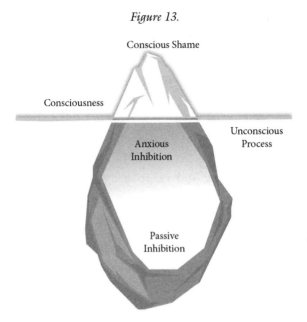

Newer psychoanalytical theory suggests that the formative dynamic is one of the socializing functions of shaming and shame that lie at the heart of the development of a sense of self. It describes the infant as living in a dream-like present until the shaming parent and its own emotional response jerks the infant into full wakefulness. In this context of early ego formation, many theoreticians speak of the shame process, with its abrupt plunge into the dissociative vagal activation, as being one of the most intensely kinesthetic feelings that we experience.

Pathological exchanges may also occur in this vital process. Unregulated parental expressions of rage and contempt evoke intense and unrelieved shame and humiliation. Shame-humiliation dynamics have been found to consistently accompany child abuse. If the stresses of the child's life are too overwhelming, paralysis in the vagally dominated state of diminished movement and interest in the environment and a general activation of the anxiety-deflation-shame state may predominate.

Glazer & Friedman suggest the formative dynamic is anchored in the right of self-expression that has been suppressed and developing primarily during the interaction between parent and child around severe early toilet training when temper tantrums were suppressed. I posit a more general origination wherein what parents let the child do for themselves and discover on their own versus what behavior they shape by giving or withdrawing their love sets the balance in children's need to please themselves versus their need to please others.

The developmental challenge is "closeness versus freedom of expression" with a basic belief that one is unappreciated and life is experienced as a "noble struggle." A "good me/ bad me" split precludes transparency in relationships, and intense internal pressure to do things "right" with a strong desire for approval predominates. Combined with an underlying distrust of further disapproval, the original sense of shame is continually reaffirmed.

The somatic holding pattern is tension in the shoulders, anus, buttocks, and thighs, with the body appearing compressed and constricted to contain and hold energy, absorbing any incoming energy that solidifies into defensive armoring. The body presents with wide or well-built shoulders and slab-like muscles, and the head tends to be set well back in the body with eyes sunk deeply in the head. The main tensions are in the flexor muscles. Energy is internalized and hypoactive, but with intellect and emotions fully integrated. Other correlates are a thick neck; pelvis tucked in; and a shortened, thick waist, often with a squashed appearance. The eyes communicate a suffering and confusion.

Figure 14 shows the body structure of a man displaying the Steadfast Supporter theme.

Figure 14.

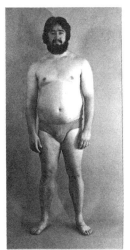 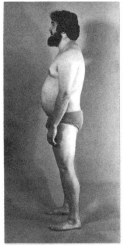

Steadfast Supportive Type

Face:	naïve expression
Neck:	short and thick
Shoulders:	tension
Back:	rounded over
Abdomen:	muscles contracted
Pelvis:	forward
Buttocks:	squeezed
Leg:	calf and thigh front underdeveloped
Feet:	tight arches
Body:	squashed; muscle-bound

The emotional presentation of the fear-based polarity of this type is one of anxiety to the point of immobilization, with feelings of guilt and shame coupled with an inability to move on from situations when needed. Closeness in relationships is accomplished through submission, and there is a likelihood of rage against rules. Anger has been turned inward, often directed at the self as guilt, and there is a fear of protesting, self-expression, and expulsion. The anal characteristics include self-deprecation and abasement and are thought to be in connection to humiliation and shame from a fear of the bottom falling out and inappropriate expression.

In the integrated state, these individuals display high levels of endurance and loyalty and have an ability to express freely while staying in connection with their own feelings. Playful and tender-hearted, they project a strong presence and excel in support roles. They also can excel in helping professions and have learned to give and express their needs in the proportions that keep themselves balanced and internally rewarded. Their anger is channeled into appropriate and direct methods of problem-solving that brings out creative resources rather than playing into a victim/persecutor/rescuer dynamic. Their warmth and receptivity put others at ease, and their competency instills trust. They are not afraid to do what needs to be done to complete tasks but do not become martyrs in the process. They have integrated a full range of emotional expression and can help others feel safe in expressing and releasing their uncomfortable feelings (e.g., shame, guilt, anger, sadness, etc.). The integrated Steadfast Supporter is a loyal and lasting friend and a true helper in the best sense of the word.

Personal Account

Rich, a musician, had strong Steadfast Supporter traits. He used the breathwork process to release repressed feelings and fear of disapproval and to renew the aliveness and innocence of his body. He was an artist with HIV who lived twenty years past this breathwork session.

"My most significant breathwork experience was my first with Jim Morningstar. I had come to Milwaukee, through the guidance of my search for Spiritual Light and the evolving circumstances of my life. I knew that my reason for coming to Milwaukee was to complete the healing of my body, mind, and soul, which had slowed down in San Francisco.

continues

"These are my recollections of my breathwork session. I remember that part of my dilemma was my inability to feel free within my body and to feel freedom through the touch of others. As I began to relax, I remember that I began to go into a very deep and dark place as my breath began to take control of my consciousness of physical breathing. I began to feel as if I were floating out into the cosmos and that I was regressing or returning to the womb. Once I was there, I felt the pressure of form coming in at me; as my conception of myself was purely mental or consciousness, I remember feeling a tremendous fear of coming out of the womb knowing that I was connected to my mother and that this could be a very serious separation. Everything was in motion, and as I began to emerge, I felt tremendous pain throughout my entire physical body. Then as I began to drift through my years of development, I would have flashes of my body registering pain through many traumas that were being administered through my mother physically and through my relatives and adults psychologically. The messages were loud and clear that touching was a bad thing and that sexual feelings were also a bad and somewhat evil thing. I guess not wanting to accept this reality is what may have kept me from going absolutely crazy, because I couldn't accept that this was the way that humans were supposed to treat each other. My body then started to become numb, and I knew that I was moving into contortions and being in positions of tetany. I remember Jim reassuring me that it was OK to feel these things and continue to breathe through them. My realization was, as Jim brought me to my awake state, that I had not really been allowing all the pain that I had experienced since birth to actually process itself through my body. It was a tremendous deep pain, as if it had even burned its way into my soul. I realized that I had been withholding love from everyone that I had ever met, because of the fear of this pain. I also realized that I was afraid of being present in my body when I touched others and was not present when others touched me.

"It was a relief that I was able to give myself permission to touch with the totality of my being and to feel all the spectrum of my feeling range that enters my body and consciousness.

"I am now able to stand firmly in my awareness and love to be loved."

BREATHWORK GOALS—STEADFAST SUPPORTER

The goal for this pattern is to heal the good/bad internal split and the ability to directly express anger. Therapeutic Breathwork goals include the following: to increase the daily sense of ease and pleasure; to enlist direct anger and decrease unconsciousness and passive-aggressive responses; to complete exhale and to release chest expansion; to support contact with creative spirit and initiative; and to decrease operating to please others at their own expense. In the integrated state, the body is solid, the personality enduring and tender. Strengths/core values include the following: a helping, compassionate, and open-hearted person who is understanding and hard-working. When working with Steadfast Supporter structure, hold the expectation that your client is not working to please *you* or taking on the role of "good girl/good boy." Be cautious of being triggered by any passive-aggressive behavior and expressing your client's anger for them. Vigorous exercise is recommended for a client to move energy, and stretching is recommended to elongate compaction. Project patience and acceptance, being sensitive not to control each client's behavior. Refrain from invading a person's privacy. Support creativity and individuality.

As a breathworker with a Steadfast Supporter structure, be mindful of the tendencies to act from an unconscious martyr role—ever trying, struggling, and suffering—under the illusion of a need to please or to be "better than" your client; to fail to see, while feeling threatened, the client's rage; and to fail to respect your need for self-care and, if necessary, a take break from breathwork when fear, depression, or your own "murderous" impulses arise. Your goals as a breathworker are to give up pretense and accept these tendencies in yourself and in others and to communicate in a straightforward manner, especially when dealing with "anger-martyr" dynamics. Your strengths as a breathworker are your acceptance and ability to endure and work through long-term issues, your supportive assistance to others, and your steadfast loyalty. Your clients will appreciate your genuine care for them.

Theme 5: Gender Balanced— Sexual Integration vs. Role Confusion

The approximate age of the emergence of the Gender Balanced structure is from the third to fifth years; when unintegrated it exemplifies the pattern of "holding on/holding in/ holding back" against the fear of falling behind or the bottom falling out. The basic right in question is, "Do I have the right to want/feel?"

Between the ages of three to six years, peak growth rates are achieved in the frontal circuits (anterior interhemispheric fiber systems) of the corpus callosum, giving rise to sustained mental vigilance and regulating the ability to plan new actions. The sex hormones underlying crucial gender differentiation are active from birth and regulated by the care-taking interactions at the onset of the oral process. Genital sensitivity and interest mature in the late practicing period. In the actual life of the toddler, elements of care-taking are interwoven with socialization, excitement, sexuality, shame inhibition, gender learning, differentiation of object relationships, and social interactions with more people and in more complex situations. Confusion with regard to gender identification and environmentally rewarded behaviors can lead to nonconforming adaptive patterns of gender identification.

Figure 15 is a simplified diagram demonstrating the complex interactions between external events, psychological interpretations, anticipation, motivation, and reward systems that involve neural connections and up or down and regulation of brain chemistry based on learning and memory. The resulting adaptive postures may reflect a compromise between environmental dictates and innate behavioral responses.

The many different views of somatic Oedipal character formation reflect this complexity. The formative dynamic is postulated to be that the expression of initiative (assertive and receptive) was hampered because of the opposite gendered parent's inability to accept emerging gender-related characteristics and through continued molding by parental expectations. This dynamic culminates in the developmental challenge of "freedom of expression versus gender identity." Lowen describes this structure as a mixture of Oedipal and preexisting Empathetic Nurturer or Steadfast Supporter character traits and results in the passive-feminine structure for males and the masculine-aggressive for females. These patterns are not defined by gender preferences as either may be adopted by hetero or homosexual orientations.

Figure 15.

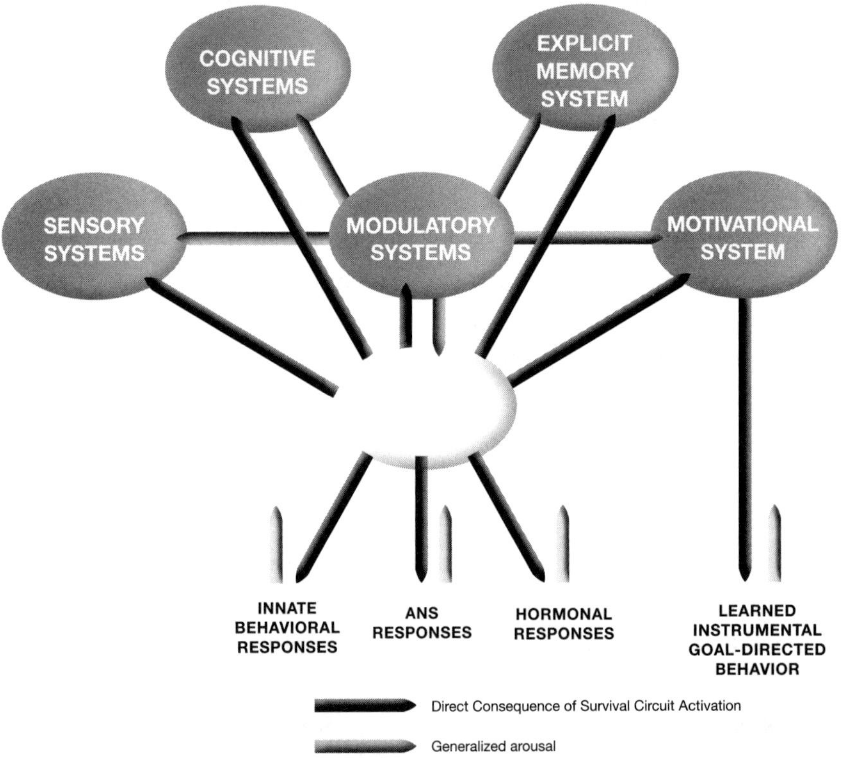
COGNITIVE SYSTEMS
EXPLICIT MEMORY SYSTEM
SENSORY SYSTEMS
MODULATORY SYSTEMS
MOTIVATIONAL SYSTEM
INNATE BEHAVIORAL RESPONSES
ANS RESPONSES
HORMONAL RESPONSES
LEARNED INSTRUMENTAL GOAL-DIRECTED BEHAVIOR
Direct Consequence of Survival Circuit Activation
Generalized arousal

The general somatic holding pattern is armoring in thighs, pelvis, chest, and eyes, but it will express differently along gender lines. Both genders demonstrate more ability to deal effectively with the world than prior body themes. In males, the physical presentation is a soft, rounded exterior, with narrow shoulders and a contracted waist with abdominal bulge. The expression is soft and compliant but with an undermining attitude when stressed, as energy is held in the head. Since expression of assertion was a threat to the father, hopelessness and despair set in and underlie his passivity as a defense against anger toward the male authority figure. This lack of aggression safeguards his fear of emotional castration by the father, but this challenge to emerging assertiveness/initiative begets a pattern of deception or compliance as the principal mode of being, masking underlying anger. The split presents in the male as one of inner feeling (male)/outer gender expression (female).

Figure 16 shows the body structure of a man with the Gender Balanced theme.

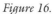

Figure 16.

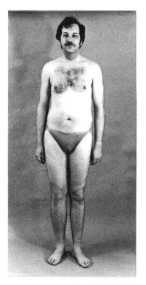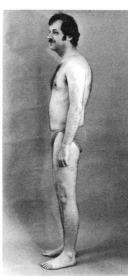

Gender-Balanced Type—Male

Face:	expressionless; soft and plastic
Shoulders:	narrow
Chest:	large breasts
Abdomen:	bulge
Hands:	soft and weak
Waist:	contracted
Movement:	never brusque or assertive
Body:	hard and rigid underneath but unified

In females, this pattern presents as a wide pelvis with narrow chest/shoulders, the lower body being weak, and with passive withholding, especially at anus. The split is expressed in the upper/lower body—the upper rigid and highly charged, lower weak and more passive—and a tightly held jaw, with sharp, focused eyes and a tendency to psychological aggression when stressed. When expressing feminine traits, the child received the parental message that it is only through strong assertion that she will be accepted. Strong pride covers a fear of dependency, as well as an ongoing struggle between strength and dependency.

Figure 17 shows the body structure of a woman with the Gender Balanced theme.

Figure 17.

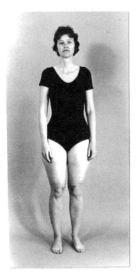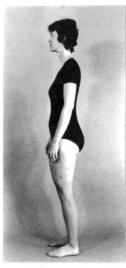

Gender-Balanced Type—Female

Upper body:	highly charged or oral
Eyes:	focused and sharp
Jaw:	forward
Lower body:	weak; passive; withholding, especially at anus; muscular
Body:	muscular development of male; excess hair; skin darker

Over-aggressiveness and competition with males is typical. Conflict between aggressive ego demands and more receptive qualities results in aggression being used in service to the ego. Ego needs such as competition and success overcome the experience of pleasure and getting one's bodily needs met. Sense of worth comes through achievement. The emotional presentation of the fear-based polarity of this type is depressive tendencies from internalized anger and underlying fear because of a block against opening up, or surrendering to, felt sensations and pleasure in the body. This pattern is noted as having impaired grounding and is prone to sudden bursts of energy, emotional expression, and dramatization of events.

In the integrated state, there is equilibrium between inner and outer states in the male and between the upper and lower states in the female. Therefore, each gender presents balanced assertion and sensitivity of both masculine and feminine attributes, without over-exaggeration of either. They accept and appropriately apply balanced male/female initiative in their work and play. They in a very real sense have the best of both worlds of receptivity and assertiveness and orchestrate the dance between them with elegance. They are comfortable with either traditional male or female roles and help bridge cultural stereotypes. Their combined male/female strengths allow them an integrative perspective that brings these talents to bear in technological as well as interpersonal problem-solving.

Personal Account

David, a hair stylist, displayed many Gender Balanced traits. He had the courage to face how his defenses built up around the lack of love from his father influenced all his subsequent relationships.

"In 1998 I met a practitioner who at the time I was seeing for colonics and reflexology. As we grew closer, breathwork came up as a next step in our work together. I was lying comfortably on a twin bed as she started drumming and chanting. I became aware of how sacred breathwork was for her and ultimately for me. I was given guidance as to how the actual breath was executed and then began my journey. I grew anxious and frightened by the way my body was reacting. I became very hot, and the gripping pain in my hands and arms was more than I thought I could endure. I voiced my concerns and was comforted by her and coached to continue breathing into the pain and tension, to stay with it—"you're doing great work." As I continued to breathe, I was confronted with the shame around my father not being able to love me. I re-experienced this great loss with the sweat rolling off my brow, mingling, and flowing into my tears. I just sobbed! How could I live unloved? My jaw was rigged with resentment. I gasped for the very breath that seemed to be torturing me. I want to end this madness and run for my life. This self-pity shifted and became one of my first visions of self-love. I realized I needed to be strong but gentle with myself. I could not give up now. I had to and wanted to live my life. I felt peace moving in and surrounding my body, embracing my raw emotion with reassurance. In that moment I saw a myriad of my life experiences flow past my mind's eye. Joined by a common thread of pain and shame, these miniature movies played on and slowly began to disappear. With the final reflection trailing off, I felt a cool breeze. My heavy, drenched, form sunk deeper into the mattress. I surrendered! With my eyelids feeling like they were turned inside

continues

out, I wept. I wept for this tiny glimpse of hope. Was I at a new beginning? I was grateful and relieved. My quivering mouth began to speak of my salvation.

"My first breathwork had blown a hole in the wall that I had built to protect me, to hide me, and to even prevent me from breathing. Through this hole I could see the light that I had been missing. With time and breath I unburied myself from the ruble of protection and separation, rebuilding a foundation that will support my future."

BREATHWORK GOALS—GENDER BALANCED

The goal for this pattern is a balanced expression of gender receptive and assertive aspects through mobilization of the split-off area/blocked energy. Therapeutic Breathwork goals include to balance inhale/exhale and assertiveness/sensitivity, to increase sense of safety in expressing sexual identity, to release jaw and pelvis, and to engage in regular belly breathing. When working with the Gender Balanced structure, guard against being threatened by the assertive female or being frustrated by the passive-aggressive male. Balancing of upper and lower/inner and outer can be supported through balancing upper energy centers with lower and between inner spiritual life and outer manifestation; cultivate assertiveness, sensitivity, directness, and equality rather than deference.

As a breathworker with a Gender Balanced structure, be mindful of the tendency as a male to express aggression indirectly, diverting it by being sweet and loving so as to be seen as a "nice guy." Your goal is to own your assertiveness so that you can promote it in your clients. As a female breathworker, there is a tendency to present a challenging "right-wrong" dynamic with males. Your goal is to integrate internal comfort with vulnerability and your feminine power. The strength of a Gender Balanced breathworker is an ability to model a blending of both masculine and feminine qualities of sensitivity and strength—head and heart.

Theme 6: Energetic Grounded—Intimacy vs. Betrayal

The approximate age of emergence of the Energetic Grounded structure is from the fourth to sixth years of life; when unintegrated it exemplifies the pattern of "holding back" against the fear of surrender to the deeper currents of life (love, sexuality, cosmic longing). The basic right in question is, "Do I have the right to love?" Neurological development all along has involved interactions among gene expression, levels of neurotransmitters, and the caregiving environment. Levels of sex hormones, which were high at birth and are decreased in middle childhood, are regulated by a caregiver's positive and negative social interactions, and they particularly underlie gender differentiation evidenced at this heightened stage of hormonal upsurge. Nurturing contact since infancy raises levels of gonadal steroids circulating in the bloodstream, unlocking genetic potential and initiating sex-linked differentiation corresponding to the dynamics described as Oedipal. A maturing sensory system in the genitals, functional since eighteen months, gives way to interest in touching and exhibiting genitalia. Pleasurable eye contact triggers excitement in the genital area and stimulated sexual self-fondling, which correspondingly occurs at the onset of the shaming interactions. Shame and regulation of sex drive are intimately connected while dyadic relationships increasingly enlarge to triadic, allowing feeling state exploration of switched intimacies through alliance with mother and then father.

The origin of the emergence of this pattern with the girl is thought to reside with the father, who gave the impression of rejecting the child's emerging sexuality—perhaps through fear of his own sexual feelings for the child. One commonly described dynamic is that one or both parents were contactful in the first years but then withdrew and diverted interest. The parents may also reject the child's feelings and desire for loving intimacy or deny the child's growing individuality and personhood. The female Energetic Grounded frozen in the fear polarity has internalized a sense of the world and of the self as one where her love and her feelings are not enough or good enough or they are too much. She is searching desperately for someone who will accept her "as she is," while simultaneously withdrawing from the deeper involvement that would make her heart vulnerable to another wounding. This is unlike the male frozen polarity of the Energetic Grounded structure who *feels* his hurt and betrayal and is identified with it. He therefore sees other people as being potentially wonderful and potentially betraying, as he struggles with his inner yearning and distrust. The developmental challenge of the Energetic Grounded pattern is "gender identity versus surrender to love."

The somatic holding pattern is a straight posture, with a shapely, tense chest and a tight, charged pelvis. The back is straight or arched, the legs are straight, and the general impression given is that of a "knight"—in either chain mail or plate armor. There is a split between heart and head. The muscular tensions are in the extensor muscles, with the strongest blocks to the flow of feelings from the heart to the genitals. The body is well-proportioned and often athletic, with adequate energy. The fear of surrender dynamically is reflected in the fear of falling (falling on one's face) with a strong, prideful, independent component. There is a tendency to be orderly and in control, although high achievement is a significant positive characteristic of this type. There can be hyperactivity with energy withheld from the core, culminating in a cold pelvis. The eyes are sparkling, bright, and present. Figure 18 shows the body structure of a man with the Energetic Grounded theme; Figure 19 shows the body structure of a woman with the Energetic Grounded theme.

Figure 18.

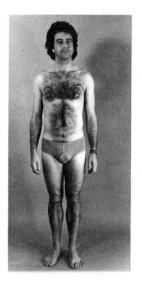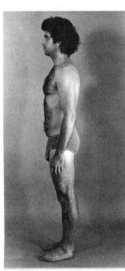

Energetic Grounded Type—Male

Face: jaw set
Eyes: bright
Shoulders: raised; squared off
Chest: out
Back: tense
Pelvis: fixed back
Body: even proportions, armored

Emotional presentation of the fear-based polarity of this type is one of anxiety (ungrounded energy). There is a fear of intimacy with a tendency to use sexuality as a form of defense against deeper feelings and commitments. A split between heart and sexuality is evidenced wherein the individual may be promiscuous or sexually active with one person while having their heart and deeper companionship with another. Often a seductive or flirtatious manner is noted with a quality of revenge that flavors actions. Type A behavioral characteristics with achievement and the need to push ahead are noted as well as injury and illness from stress because of the need to be on top and in the lead.

Figure 19.

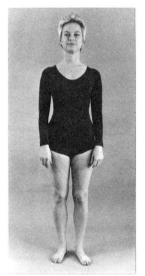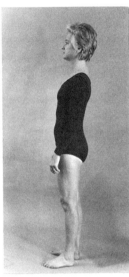

Energetic Grounded Type—Female

Face:	tight; jaw tense
Neck:	base of skull; extreme tension
Shoulders:	immobile
Lower back:	tight
Pelvis:	pulled back; soft; sexually alive
Legs:	stiff
Upper body:	rigid
Lower body:	soft; yielding

The integrated state of the Energetic Grounded theme is one of attractiveness and alertness, in other words, a capable and healthy individual who is able to deal with challenges from strength and focus. High-energy, they possess directness and connection with others and are able to hold both sensual and heart-centered energy. They can surrender to loving feelings and maintain long-term intimate relationships. Their ability to both be grounded and open to surrender favor their success in many areas of life. They bring a full complement of life energy to whatever they undertake and are able to enlist a wide range of resources through their personal magnetism. Hence, they can take on great challenges without needing the adrenaline rush or great drama of their unintegrated states. They are now able to balance achievement with heartfelt satisfaction in relationship.

Personal Account

John, a parole officer and counselor, showed Energetic Grounded features including his rigid chest and fear of letting his heart out, while engaging in a challenging occupation. His breathwork exemplified the physical and emotional confines in which he felt trapped.

"I was determined, with my third breathwork, to remember and be conscious of what I experienced. I started breathing, with Ric, my therapist, offering me encouragement. After ten to fifteen minutes of continuous breathing, I began experiencing myself trapped between four walls. The walls were tall and smooth, and I could not climb over them. There were no openings of any kind, so I could not pass through them. But, I knew I had to get through them, so I continually walked/ran into the walls hoping I could get through. As I kept this up, my frustration grew.

"All of a sudden, I was aware someone was behind me, and I became frightened. I did not want to turn around, but I found myself doing it anyway. It was dark, and I could not quite make out who it was, but I knew it was someone familiar to me. I realized he had a gun in his hand and was pointing it at me. I stood frozen in confusion and terror. I heard him laugh and saw him pull the trigger. The momentary flash of the gun illuminated his face, and I saw it was me. As the bullet struck me, I began to dissolve with the laughter echoing in my mind.

"My body and walls dissolved, and I began to experience who I am beyond the pretense, the body, the ego, my armor. I began experiencing who I really am. It was a wonderfully free, joyous, and moving experience. I remember crying, tears streaming joyously down my face as I experienced more and more of me. And then, suddenly I began dissolving again. I became momentarily frightened as I felt myself being drawn into something bigger. Bigger than myself, I was an insignificant speck in some vast consciousness/God. After my initial fear, I began breathing into the experience, feeling greater and greater joy. I felt love, immense, and unqualified love. Love so strong, yet so safe, I felt swathed in it like a baby. Love coming from all sources and directed toward me yet not just me. It was total and complete love directed everywhere. And then, that too, dissolved, and I became aware of my body, my tears, and Ric."

BREATHWORK GOALS—ENERGETIC GROUNDED

The goal for the Energetic Grounded pattern is to experience being loved and appreciated for one's self and to relax and play in order to experience real contact with others. Therapeutic Breathwork goals include the following: to integrate inhale and exhale, softening the armoring; to unite love and sexuality; and to feel safe being vulnerable with others.

When working with the Energetic Grounded structure, be careful of the context projected, which is not competitive, jealous, or one based on becoming friends or intimate. Journaling as a tool of self-discovery is recommended, as is examination of assumptions about relationships. Stress forgiveness when appropriate and self-acceptance. Work toward emotional release of betrayal and grief, and facilitate inner child and codependency work. Provide patience, with an open heart; while dealing with challenges, the client may defend against letting go into their feelings. Project gentle, trustworthy support for the vulnerable feelings as they emerge. Understand that underneath the prickly defense system is deep hurt.

As a breathworker with an Energetic Grounded structure, be mindful of the tendency, as a male, to unconsciously withhold your heart in an effort to be safe or to compete, holding back your love under the illusion that you are a misunderstood yet loving person. Your goal is to give up and soften in your ability to trust the boundaried closeness between yourself and your client. As a female breathworker, your tendency may be to withhold your heart out of pride and determination and, like an unrecognized princess, expect your commands to be obeyed. Your goal is to let go and step down from any pedestal and meet your client on the same level. The strengths of the Energetic Grounded breathworker are your strong energetic contact, your ability to model self-confidence and success to clients, and your ability to engage in effective partnerships.

Conclusion

Broadly speaking, the first two of the six body themes, Psychic Sensitive and Empathetic Nurturing, have challenges with their inhale, taking in a full complement of life energy. The second two body themes, Inspirational Leader and Steadfast Supportive, have their major challenges with their exhale, releasing and letting go of their holding patterns. The last two, Gender Balanced and Energetic Grounded, have their challenges with the integration of their inhale and exhale, balancing their yin and yang, male and female energies.

What I have presented in this chapter is an introduction to the use of breath and body theme awareness and tools to free chronic holding patterns. No one is defined by a body theme, and there is no theme cookbook for self-realization. Nonetheless, the art and science of Therapeutic Breathwork, combined with body-theme awareness and used as an adjunct to an individual's own power to heal and grow, has been one of the most incisive and effective tools I have seen people use and adapt to their own needs. The simple yet effective gifts we all have as human beings—our breath, our loving intention, our authentic movement, and self-expression—all come together to inspire people to find their own source and heart-centered path in life.

I see this growing field of mind-body-spirit work as a critical counterbalance to our technological evolution. Daily discoveries in clinical practice and the neurosciences underscore the importance of honoring our bodies as wondrous storehouses of past wisdom and current potential for our next stage of evolution. It is through a renewed spirit of interdisciplinary sharing and cooperation that we are recovering our wholeness.

Therapeutic Breathworker training has been undertaken by practitioners in all the major healing professions. They have adopted the heightened breath awareness, sensitivity, and expressiveness that this training involves to their own healing practices, from medical arts such as physical and occupational therapy, anesthesiology, dentistry, massage, and energy medicine to psychotherapy and counseling. I invite you to contribute your personal and professional expertise to this evolving field of healing and transformation.

In the next and final chapter, you will look at applications of breathwork in daily life, professional practice, and personal growth.

Chapter 6

Therapeutic Breathwork's Application in Life Challenges, Professional Practice, and Conscious Growth

I am never alone wherever I am. The air itself supplies me with a century of love. When I breathe in, I am breathing in the laughter, tears, victories, passions, thoughts, memories, existence, joys, moments, and the hues of the sunlight on many tones of skin; I am breathing in the same air that was exhaled by many before me. The air that bore them life. And so how can I ever say that I am alone?

—C. JOYBELL C.

As with most healing and personal development techniques, people come to Therapeutic Breathwork originally looking for something they think they do not have in their lives (relief from pain, ennui, or anxiety) or an inner sense there is something more for them and they are ready to have it. If it is one of these precipitants or depression, confusion, or overwhelm, the initial breathwork sessions often open the doors for new life energy on the cellular level and provide a breakthrough from the prison of their minds and hearts. These sessions, even if they are painful, provide a ray of hope in the seemingly bleak landscape of their life. It is exciting if not exhilarating in many instances. If the sessions are progressing well, clients soon learn that each session is different and to suspend the mental expectations that try to recapture what has gone before. This provides even greater joy in that what is being learned is not a formula to be applied to every life situation but a set of tools to take into each challenge with which to be creative and empowering.

There then comes the time when the storehouse of past trauma, incomplete relationships, and holding patterns have been significantly reduced, such that the ecstatic fireworks of the original sessions have subsided. It is here that many think their time with breathwork has come to an end. Indeed, that may be true for many whose purpose was to address specific troubled areas of their life.

But for many others, it is only the beginning of a much greater adventure. Certainly the miracle of ongoing contentment and the use of breathwork as a regular maintenance tool is a logical next step. Not only do I endorse this, but I have practiced some form of breathwork daily for this purpose since the mid-1970s. Beyond this, however, is the use of breathwork for exploration and growth, charting new waters in the ocean of unlimited possibilities. Pioneers in the field of using breathwork for personal and planetary growth have left the realms of consensus reality and explored the worlds of spontaneous remission of diseases, spiritual enlightenment, and physical immortality. It is not the purview of this book to look at each of these in detail but to inspire the continued use of breathwork beyond the mind's original agenda of alleviating suffering to callings of the spirit toward a deeper embracing of who we are beyond our ideas and fixed identities.

Some choose to have guidance on these explorations and will select an appropriate professional or a person experienced in journeying with nonordinary states of consciousness. Someone who is familiar with the use of breathwork is recommended but not always necessary if experienced in dealing with altered states. In fact, you may end up teaching them about the use of breath to reach these altered states that they have not previously witnessed. When Stan Grof, MD, could no longer obtain official permission to conduct therapy with LSD, it prompted him to explore the shamanistic techniques that used breath to induce trance. He found ancient traditions that employed breath as a means to achieve states of knowingness outside of the logical rational side of the brain. These states that the shaman used to initiate healing processes are similar to states clients use to open doors physically, emotionally, mentally, and spiritually to heal themselves. I have been privileged to witness this over the decades.

I generally do not tout the seemingly miraculous healing I have seen in breathwork, like the young woman who incurred the wrath of her surgeon. She came in for a presurgery breathwork session and then during the surgery the doctor found there were no longer any fibroids to operate on when she was opened up. These stories can prompt people to use breathwork as a panacea to cure everything. More to the point, breathwork is a tool to open our awareness to all the levels of our being and effect a greater healing of restoring wholeness that may have little to do with alleviating symptoms. In some cases, coming to forgiveness over a past abortion or even an abortion attempt on a client before their birth might be a greater healing than a spontaneous fibroid removal. Indeed, I consider some of the greatest miracles that happen in breathwork or anywhere a "change of heart" that may not be recorded by anyone outside of the person affected, but that profoundly changes the course of their history and consequently all those around them. That is why even though I always recommend having a conscious intention in going into a session, I also add the *cosmic clause*, "This or something greater." In other words, I always let my conscious intention defer to something greater that my higher self may have in store for me.

What follows are stories I have selected to illustrate how people have used breathwork to deal with life challenges, as a professional in their practice, or for conscious growth. These three categories often overlap, as you will see in reading them. They are meant to inspire courage and creativity in the application of breathwork.

Life Challenges

Remember to breathe. It is, after all, the secret of life.

—GREGORY MAGUIRE, *A Lion Among Men*

Life Challenges Account #1

Lani, a healing practitioner, followed her intuition in asking for a breathwork session with the right practitioner, which helped her to release a pervasive feeling of not being helped in life and to improve her breathing.

"One day I intuitively knew that it would be wise to do breathwork that day with Catherine Rose, a nurse breathworker. I didn't know why. We had previously discussed exchanging sessions, and it just hadn't manifested. This particular day I was assertive in that I was to be the breathwork recipient, and this was that day.

continues

"She had me start with color flowing through my chakras and twenty fast-paced, connected breaths.

"Soon I found myself back to the time when I was four years of age, at a family picnic, and hit in the face full-force in the nose by circular swings. At the time, there was no one there to help me. I heard the crush of my bones and smelled blood. I was terrified. This time there was Catherine Rose, a registered nurse. She helped me. She was there. I was so very extremely grateful. I held on to her and cried over and over, "I needed a nurse." Time was transcended, and Catherine Rose gave me what I needed back then.

"I smelled blood for a few days afterward and then found that my nose and breathing had improved from how it had been prior to this breathwork session."

Life Challenges Account #2

Jennifer, a retail presentation coordinator, translated her practice of breathwork from therapy into a daily self-monitoring device that is there for her in times of heightened stress.

"Breathwork has become an invaluable healing tool through therapy and into my everyday life. What it helped me realize was that talk therapy only did not allow the full experience of my emotions. Experiencing, not just talking out emotions, taps into a whole new dimension for healing.

"My first experience was in a group setting, but what I have found that furthered my growth the most was paired breathwork. I worked with a certified breathworker to practice monthly. I moved from a place of fear to living my dreams. Using breathwork as a monthly practice helped unlock the emotions trapped in my body and work through what was brought up in a session.

"I draw on this practice daily to quickly check in on my emotional state. It's almost an immediate reaction if I am holding my breath and take a minute to take a deep breath. It's such an important practice in my life that recently after I had my first child and was buying my first home and experiencing stress, several family members and coworkers asked if I had breathed recently. I found an opportunity to breathe with a group that next weekend."

Life Challenges Account #3

Pat, a psychotherapist, used breathwork to release longstanding resent-
ment and abandonment themes. This not only cleared emotional baggage
from the past but opened doors to more gratitude and fulfillment in her
present life and work.

"My most significant breathwork took place on my daughter's seven-teenth birthday. I went into the session a little heavy-hearted because I was participating in a weekend breathwork retreat away from home and I would not see my daughter on her birthday.

"I was twenty-seven years old when I gave birth to my daughter. She was born in a hospital in Richmond, Virginia. Although I had taken natural childbirth classes, I opted for epidural anesthesia in my fourteenth hour of labor. She was born using low forceps at 1 a.m. and was ten days late. I was terrified to give birth, and although my husband was with me, our relationship had been strained for some time. This was my first time in the hospital as a patient, and I was also scheduled to stay on for a thyroidec-tomy following the birth.

"As I began the conscious connected breathing, I had many visual images come up. I could see my large belly and swollen breasts, and all through the session I was aware of the image of a mature woman's eye, watching me closely and waiting…. I did not recognize the 'eye,' but it was not intimidating. I felt tingling sensations up and down my right side. I 'felt' my water break and the warm sensation of fluid rushing down my thighs. I 'tasted' a foul taste in my mouth. I experienced the need to 'push' and felt my body bear down against the mat in preparation for birth. Then waves of voracious hunger come over me. It made me very distracted and wanting to search for food. My partner encouraged me to stay with the breath, and with her assistance, I was able to stay focused.

"I was very 'altered' as I continued to breathe but also very aware that I was supported. I felt surrounded by 'love.' It also felt as if one of my supporters were at my feet, assisting me to rid myself of the negative emotions associated with this very difficult time in my life. At the time of the birth I was primarily dealing with the fear associated with giving birth, the

continues

fear of an upcoming surgery, and the fear of my husband's erratic mood shifts. Years later, as I 'rebirth,' I was grieving the loss of my marriage eight months after the birth of my daughter due to the tragic circumstances surrounding my husband's complete shift.

"The waves of sadness continued to come for what felt like hours: the sadness was not connected to any specific thought; it just felt like a 'release' of emotion that I had been carrying for years.

"Following the release, my partner who was assisting me with the breathwork seemed 'far away.' I no longer felt her presence next to me. In the 'real' birth, my husband actually walked out of the delivery room soon after my daughter was born. In the rebirth, anger immediately came up within me. I also felt a very old feeling of being encouraged to 'let my guard down, only to be abandoned.' Later I found out that my partner did indeed move out of my field and sat next to the wall, allowing me the space to integrate my hard work in silence. I never asked for her but suffered silently, which to this day is my pattern. I realized later that this time, however, the hurt I felt was tempered by the adult in me that 'knew better—that if my partner did leave, it was for a good reason, and I can be assured that she was not far away.'

"In the days following the exquisite breathwork experience, I came to forgive my husband for the pain and abandonment I had felt for years. I even love him now so much more. I love him every day for giving me Sara, for Sara has given me so much comfort, love, and pride. She shines with his intelligence, his compassion, his humanitarian character, and gentle spirit. I have come to really value all of the other special gifts he brought into my life, including the love of the outdoors and golden retrievers, most especially, for being one of my supporters in helping me develop and grow into what I am today. For without him and Sara, I would not have been on this particular path that has led me to God (and love) through the breath."

Life Challenges Account #4

Laurie, a housing manager and artist, used breathwork to face her anxiety, overcome a phobia, and assist her husband while he was going through a heart attack.

"I was very frightened when I first did breathwork. Emotions came up that I didn't know how to deal with. I'm a very controlling person, and letting myself feel the emotions was very difficult. I've never been in that state of relaxation before. I would shut down in the middle of breathwork although in time I realized it helped me become aware of my inner issues. Focusing on my breath helped me relax, and it allowed me to focus on any emotions that would arise and become more in tune with my inner self. I would then make a plan on how to approach my healing process. It was usually with my art. The healing process may even have included breathwork.

"One of the reasons why I started using breathwork was for my anxiety. I had it for five-plus years. Between breathwork and quite a bit of counseling it would never go away. Finally one day I realized it was gone. I think I gave into it rather than it controlling me. Today I am anxiety-free.

"I still use breathwork when I get scared. I even had my husband using it when he had his heart attack in the emergency room. He's having all sorts of doctors around him in the emergency room, and I'm standing next to him having him focus on his breath and follow my rhythm.

"I also used breathwork when I had to take pain pills from a surgery. I had a phobia of pills because I didn't want to feel out of control. I was afraid to feel high. When I finally had to take the pills just recently, I did breathwork and focused on my fear. I somehow realized that it was OK to feel high if you are in pain. It took a few days to get over the fear once I started with the pain pills. I did some breathwork to help me focus on that fear, and it calmed me down. Now my fear is gone. Or maybe I was just in so much pain that I wanted the pain pills. Regardless, I'm over this phobia that I've had for over fifteen years."

Life Challenges Account #5

Thomas, a hypnotherapist, had a significant release of early life trauma during a breathwork session that not only brought relief from the memories and feeling he was harboring and its influence on his relationships but also gave him insight that was useful in his professional career.

"A way breathwork enhanced the counseling process for me is by relieving, in one breathwork therapy session, the emotional trauma from a childhood incest incident. It was an incident I had brought up and spoken about in therapy to various counselors over the years but prior to this breathwork experience had never realized just how powerfully it had affected my child's consciousness back then.

"I had had no intention or expectation of summoning up trauma but was willing to try out a technique still fairly new to me with a therapist I knew, respected, and trusted.

"I had done one breathwork session with a facilitator several decades earlier, in the 1970s when rebirthing/breathwork was just emerging, and it had been essentially a pleasurable experience.

"However, as I went through the process this time I suddenly re-experienced, as the child I had been, the terror, shame, and fear I had felt. 'I knew it was wrong,' I heard the child say.

"Aided by my compassionate facilitator, I achieved a cathartic healing. One appointment, one time was enough. I came back for another appointment later and also did breathwork on my own several times at home, but no further 'lodged' emotions about the incident came up to be released.

"The power of the experience led me to research the specific effects of incest between various family combinations. I found the effects of sister victimizing brother to be consistent with what I felt during my re-experience of the incest event."

Professional Application

Breath is the bridge which connects life to consciousness, which unites your body to your thoughts. Whenever your mind becomes scattered, use your breath as the means to take hold of your mind again.

—THICH NHAT HANH, *The Miracle of Mindfulness: An Introduction to the Practice of Meditation*

Many professionals have adopted breathwork to their practices. This has been particularly heartwarming to me. I highly encourage the creative adaptations of the principles and techniques of breathwork to other healing arts. I find that this adds to the power and effectiveness of both breathwork and the various healing arts to which it has been applied. The Spirit of Breath cannot be confined to one form or one set of techniques. It is my dream that the principles and healing power of the breath be more consciously applied to all healing arts and the mastery of everyday life. Here are just a few examples of this creative application.

Professional Application Account #1

Jayne, a massage therapist and Therapeutic Breathworker, incorporates her training as a professional breathworker with her expertise as a massage therapist. As with most professionals, she uses her discretion as to when and how to apply these tools, taking cues and feedback from each client.

"I have worked with many survivors of trauma over the past twenty years. In the past thirteen years I have utilized the tool of breathwork. I've been astonished at the impact of the breath on individual and group processes. It has helped so many of the clients with whom I have partnered in their healing journeys to reconnect with their bodies. I am thrilled by what I have seen as it brings hope to those who have experienced severe trauma. Many have exited their bodies as a way to protect themselves from the trauma through which they were surviving.

continues

"In my experience with breathwork I have seen and personally experienced it to be a gentle and at the same time powerful tool in helping people to bypass strong mental, emotional, physical, and spiritual barriers to healing. I've seen individuals begin to trust themselves again after such a vast disconnect from their very source. Then I have witnessed clients slowly awakening and reconnecting the frozen or forgotten pieces of themselves.

"'Marta' came to me for therapeutic massage at the recommendation of her counselor. Two years prior to entering my therapy room she had left her second abusive marriage. With her therapist she had done some deep and powerful emotional and mental healing of the abuse that she had lived through in childhood as well as in the marriages. Marta came to me to address some of the physical repercussions from the forty-plus years of trauma. She had constant headaches and backaches. Her body felt tense and was held in a protective stance.

"After four sessions of massage, Martha stated that her headaches had gone away. Her backaches remained. The pain coursed up and down her spine. As Marta entered the room for her fifth session, I was running behind and still had the breathwork mat on the floor. I greeted her and apologized for the delay. She inquired about the floor mat. I explained that it was used for breathwork and then described breathwork. She looked intrigued, so I offered a breathwork session instead of a massage. She accepted the offer and experienced her first breathwork session. I did not see Marta again until two weeks later. When she returned, she said to me, 'You know the breathwork session we did last time? It cleared 80 percent of the back pain that I have been having for years, and it hasn't returned!' I was just as amazed as she was and thrilled that her courage led to such a powerful healing experience.

"Breathwork helps each of us to become more connected with our deepest source and allows us to really live more fully, no matter what walk of life we are navigating. Breathwork can help us to gain more clarity as we discover our life purpose, create peaceful conflict resolutions, navigate next steps along our path, and deepen our relationships. As a practitioner, breathwork has helped me to develop a compassionate connection and healing partnership between clients and myself without negating important professional boundaries. Personally it has given me much confidence, clarity, and a deep sense of peace as I walk my path in life."

Professional Application Account #2

Michelle, an experienced physical therapist, found, during an advanced Craniosacral Therapy Training, her experience as a breathworker to be exactly what was needed to help her training colleague be more receptive to her own healing work.

"Nancy was in my group and was terrified of being touched and worked with. She had endured severe emotional and physical abuse (especially around and in her mouth and face) by her parents.

"When Nancy was the lead therapist, she became very controlling—even obnoxious—directing who to work where, telling us what specific techniques to use, and not allowing each of us to blend our unique work with each other, which was ultimately what happened as we got to know each other and as we became more adept at reading energy (our patient's energy as well as each other's). This didn't happen when Nancy was in charge.

"On the flip side, when Nancy was the patient, she was also in control, telling who to touch her where and how much pressure to apply when. Actually, she was very good at it!

"That afternoon, it was my turn to be the lead therapist for Nancy. I was very apprehensive. Nancy lay on her back, and I allowed my team to choose where they wanted to be. I decided to work at Nancy's head and shoulders. I gently placed my hands on her shoulders (I sat at the head of the table, behind her head). Everyone then gently laid their hands on Nancy. After a few minutes, we all began to sense the craniosacral rhythm. Very soon, her body began to let us in deeper and then she decided to 'put on the brakes'—giving directions, telling us where to go, etc. I remember myself beginning to feel unnerved, and I had to work so hard at staying grounded physically as well with my purpose.

"I very slowly told her how much we all loved her and how much we all wanted to work with her; however, this required a level of trust on her part. I also told her that we were not going to become her servants during her session on the table and that we were going to help guide her with whatever she needed to do and that she was not going to direct the session with her head; otherwise, we would stop. An interesting thing happened next, something that I have never felt before: Nancy could control

continues

her craniosacral rhythms! The rhythm is generally used as a 'truth' signal. The rhythm will 'tell' you if the conscious message or physical sensation is true, but Nancy could change it to serve her needs! I was at a loss for a moment, until ... I realized that she was hardly breathing. So, I decided to facilitate her breathing, and then everything slowly changed.

"Connected breathing was the hardest and most valuable assignment for Nancy. It took constant coaching on my part. We worked for at least thirty minutes on breathing, and as she stayed with it, her ribcage began to soften, allowing more physical pain to surface and be felt. It was an amazing experience to feel. I had to keep grounding myself, until after ninety minutes, I was exhausted, and I asked my teacher for help. It wasn't until then that Nancy allowed our teacher to do some intra-oral (mouth) work. It was wonderful to watch! Nancy released a lot of pain and fear and slowly opened to beginning to trust another again.

"I felt such gratitude to be able to facilitate our group with helping Nancy. She was a teacher for all of us."

Professional Application Account #3

Teri, a licensed counselor, has the following degrees: MEd, Licensed Professional Counselor, Clinical Substance Abuse Counselor, Licensed School Counselor, Reiki Master, Energy Practitioner, and Breathworker. She works as a therapist with Native Americans and is a shaman. She has adapted breathwork into every facet of her trainings.

"The joy of sharing breathwork with others on a professional and personal level has brought many gifts into my life. One of the many gifts has been being able to connect with another person's spiritual essence or soul. Through these connections, I have been able to dialogue with the soul and facilitate energetic healing on many levels.

"Michael came to see me because he was experiencing anxiety and having panic attacks that scared him and greatly reduced his ability to recover after having one. He also wanted to calm the constant chatter and racing thoughts that were always moving through his mind. While

continues

working with Michael, we were able to discover the origin of his anxiety. As a young boy he was able to recall the trauma he experienced within his family system. The negative energy seemed to settle in his sacral chakra and was blocking his third-eye chakra. Michael set the intention that he wanted to breathe for releasing and relaxation.

"As we began to breathe together on a consistent basis, I noticed he was able to allow his physical body to relax so his energetic body could release and begin to heal. During one of our sessions, as we were breathing, I unwound and opened his sacral and third eye chakras. I placed one of hands directly underneath his chest, at the back of the heart, and the other on the front of his chest, over his heart. I held my hands there and began to gently massage as I dialogued with his soul. I reassured his soul that it was safe, loved, and OK for it to release the hurt and the negative energy it stored.

"The conversation lasted less than three minutes. The client said he felt an incredible sense of warmth, and a surge moved through him and exit through the top of his head. I could feel my own body gently quiver as that release took place. The client continued to breathe and release until his breath was slow, extended, and relaxed.

"The impact of that particular session was profound for Michael as he released the energy of his childhood trauma, reclaimed a piece of his soul, and was able to eliminate his panic attacks through the use of his own breath."

Conscious Growth

"In our breath lies not only the gift of life, but also the basis of all resolutions, ideas, and infinite audacity."

—DR. JACINTA MPALYENKANA

Stories of transcendental experiences while doing breathwork are legion. The nonordinary state of consciousness that often happens during sessions does open the doors of awareness that may include other levels and dimensions of our being. My primary interest in what happens during a session, however, is its relevance to the present life of the client. Just to have a litany of altered experiences is not necessarily useful and in fact may become a distraction from the business at hand (i.e., present life fulfillment). When a "past life" or transcendent experience takes place during a session, I believe integration of the relevance of it into one's current life is of primary importance. This is the job of the breathworker, not to be a "wet blanket" on the client's elevated state but to help them translate that highness into an overall life elevation, rather than a special "high" to be sought as an escape from their current life. This may not feel immediately as glamorous as reinforcing specialness, which unfortunately can all too easily translate to separation in "being above" or "different than" others. The messages from these experiences are not always easily or immediately put into logical "to do's." Nor should we try to interpret our clients' experiences to fit our paradigm of healing or growth. Helping our clients ground and have some support in integrating their experiences over the ensuing weeks after the session may take no more than letting them know we are available to talk or may involve follow-up work even sooner than a scheduled appointment. I will give them potential ways of holding their experience if they are confused or ungrounded and are looking for some reference point from which to move forward. This could be a simple as "Feeling ungrounded for a while can happen when you are expanding the awareness of your ground of being," to a more detailed reference such as "Your intention at the onset of the session was to release your sense of stuckness, and you seem to have opened the doors to a much greater energy flow that may take a bit to relax into." In other words, my role as a facilitator is sometimes to be a reflector of my clients' overall process while they are in the middle of change.

The following are a few examples of nonordinary experiences that range from images of this lifetime to what might seem "otherworldly." In each of these accounts, the clients were able to integrate the energy of their experiences into present-life empowerment.

Conscious Growth Account #1

Kathy, a mortgage officer, had a strong intention to learn from her birth process and took that into the breathwork retreat. One could try to discount her experiences as a product of auto-suggestion. My experience, however, of being present during the overwhelmingly intense physical enactments of birth and the subsequent changes in the thinking, feeling, and acting of the participants (including myself) over the years leads me to conclude a) the nervous system is reenacting sensations and memories beyond the pale of conscious memory and b) even if some measure of auto-suggestion were to be a component of the reenactment, the results on one's life and relationships coming out give consensual validation to the process.

"For several months prior to the July breathwork workshop I began thinking regularly about my birth process and how that might have impacted my personality and my life. I knew I had been held back for at least twenty minutes as they held my mother's legs together until the doctor arrived. I couldn't seem to stop thinking about it, so I decided to dedicate the weekend to exploring my birth.

"I began the process of this exploration well before the weekend, at least two weeks before so I was ready to breathe on it when I arrived at Transformations. My intention that session was to experience my birth and obtain any pertinent information that would help me to understand myself better and to be more fully alive.

"The session began much like any other session: breathing to get into the rhythm and to let go so I could go as deep as possible. It was nice at first; I felt free and light and happy. Shortly after the session began, I could feel pain around my head as if a band was placed completely around the circumference of my forehead. I could see the color purple/violet associated with the pain. It got stronger and stronger until I felt as if my head would burst. I breathed into it and realized that it was my head crowning from my mother's body and also where they stopped me from emerging. I kept my breath going into that painful band surrounding my head.

continues

"Soon I felt confined, and I had the urge to push my way out. It was dark and tight, and my head was killing me. I tried frantically to get out, but pushing with my hands and feet in attempts to free myself was fruitless. I tried until I reached the point of exhaustion. I had to rest. I had to regain my strength to try again.

"When I felt strong enough, I tried again to get free. I struggled and even tried to turn around to see if that would work, I pushed and I shoved, and I began to feel a sense of panic and deep rage. The harder I tried to free myself, the angrier I became. Nothing seemed to work. I was trapped. I realized that I couldn't breathe, and I started to feel sheer terror; just then the doctor arrived.

"On the third try, I emerged from my mother's body, and although I still felt the anger and perhaps resentment, I also felt complete and utter joy surrounding the freedom. I could breathe again! For a long while I was exhausted and just needed to rest. I had made it! The struggle was over.

"As I lay there processing, I realized that the only other time I had felt that anger was when my father tried to hold me back. I think I associated my birth anger with my dad, and it probably played a major role in our relationship as a child and teenager. I also realized that the challenge I experienced during birth has been familiarly repeated over and over again as I have chosen challenging people and situations throughout my life.

"That night after class, the process continued, and when I awoke on Saturday, my head still hurt, my sinuses and ears were plugged up, and my throat was on fire. My body had taken on all these physical signs that surely followed my birth almost fifty years ago. I was totally amazed by this.

"As I continued to process, I realized another life pattern I have taken on is to go, go, go until I can't go anymore. I am sure that I got that from the struggle to be born and am happy to know I can let go of it now. I also realized that the strong need I have for freedom comes from this birth experience.

"On a more positive note, the positives I got from this experience have impacted my life deeply. One of them is that I am not afraid of hard, challenging work; I even thrive on it sometimes. I was also empowered as I worked toward my goal of freedom that has contributed to my self-esteem

continues

and self-confidence. It definitely contributed for my love of life and the inherent joy I have always felt underlying every other emotion. It taught me to fight for what I want, to not give up, and that determination pays off. Most importantly I believe that this experience created my deep passion for the life and the world. My passion has been my life force, and I also learned that patience will always lead to my highest and best.

"This experience has definitely been one of the highlights of my life. It confirms how powerful and beneficial breathwork can be. It also made me aware of how important it is to go back to the birth process to determine the impact it has had upon my life. I am very surprised how twenty minutes could have impacted my life in all the ways it has. I will now be able to assist other breathers in their birth experiences when they are ready. A most amazing experience.

"On Saturday's session I took what I had processed, the gifts that I had received, and incorporated them at a cellular level. I feel as though my life has been changed for the better from this experience. In the water on Saturday, I was able to redo the birth, learn about what I needed to change to come back into the world letting go of the things that have negatively impacted my life, and hold onto those that have been positives. I really feel like I can let go of those old patterns that have not served me well. I can move forward as a positively changed and more well-rounded person who can make a definite impact upon the world and those I will assist in the future. "

Conscious Growth Account #2

Matthew, a young psychotherapist, was taking his first breathworker training. What he experienced during one of his first sessions could be interpreted from many points of view (e.g., an imaginary visualization to help his body release, a past life experience, an archetypical struggle of human collective consciousness, etc.). He preferred to call it "connecting to the primal self," which he felt most empowering and relevant to his current needs. This is not an end point in his growth but an important step along the way.

continues

"Sitting in training class listening to a lecture before we go into a breathing session, I noticed the back of my neck was tight and the point where my spine joins the base of my skull hurt. It was getting really bad and moved to the point of pain. To me, these sensations indicated a huge headache was about to happen. I have been told these are tension headaches and other sorts of interesting theories. So for the next breathing session, I wanted to go into these pain points and discover for myself what this was about.

"The class moved outside, and my partner and I found a great spot under a tree with a large grassy area. I stated my intention to explore this pain in my neck and skull to my breathworker and proceeded to drop into a very fast circular breath. As I moved my neck to stretch out the left side, I had this visual flash of a man holding my neck to the side and slamming a ramrod down through side of my neck along my spine. This ramrod went all the way to the base of my spine and was very painful. I was being restrained, and I had this sense I was being 'made an example of.' As I continued to breathe, the sensations in my body released. I had a very similar experience on the right side of my neck when I stretched it, finding another ramrod to the base of my spine. There was a sensation that this was some sort of torture as I was still alive but immobile and in lots of pain. As I continued to breathe, the energies released, and only the pain left was at the base of my skull. This pain was excruciating. My body felt like it wanted to go into the fetal position, and I went with it. There in the fetal position in the grass, I felt a spike driven into the base of my skull. I knew this spike was the death stroke. My fear of death came to the surface as well as sadness for I had done nothing to deserve this. There in the fetal position I cried as I could feel my life draining away into nothing.

"For thirty days before this professional breath training, I had been doing thirty minutes of circular breathing every day. I have worked through many emotional releases and had gained a trust with the Spirit of Breath to hold me so long as I returned to the breath. In the grass weeping my death, I found my breath and returned to the circular breathing. The base of my skull felt open and pain-free. I had regained some calm when the breathworker mentioned something; I do not know what he said but knew it was not right for me. I responded, 'No, I will stand on my own two feet.'

continues

And I stood up. There was freedom in my body and joyousness, a liberation. I felt strength return to my body and proudly extended both middle fingers, 'F___ you, mother f___ers, I am still here.'

"My legs seemed to want to move, and I began to bounce ever so slightly. There in my pocket a jingle happened. A shit-eating grin came over my face. Upon waking up this morning, I had slipped the buffalo horn claws my wife gave me for my fortieth birthday into my pocket, and in the other pocket I had my four-chambered heart medicine pouch. I wonder if I can get that jingle louder? So I danced and spun around, all the time listening to the buffalo horns in my pocket clack together. I dropped to all fours and hopped around. Leaning low, I smelled the ground, and a very 'primal' energy emerged in my body. I continued to hop, and at some point I did a forward roll. Eventually, I laid in the grass drinking in the sunshine. My mind wandered back to the absurdity of someone trying to 'make an example' of someone else. Laughter emerged deep within my belly. Laying there in the grass, I laughed and laughed. I do not know how long I laughed, but it was delightful.

"A few days have passed, and I look at this session with different eyes. Educational, work, and community institutions have tried to make me fit into their models throughout my life. Anything outside of the normal is frowned upon. Through shaming and other methods, these institutions have tried to shape me to fit the 'norm' and have used me as the example. Ultimately this type of treatment deeply wounded my soul. But the absurdity of the whole thing is you cannot kill a soul. You can wound it, but a person has the resiliency built into them to bounce back. My body feels more fluid, and my spine is free to move again. I have my freedom of expression. 'F___ you, mother f___ers, I am still here.'"

Conscious Growth Account #3

Kesha, a massage therapist and breathworker, reveals a series of life-altering synchronicities initiated by her breathwork process that went from personal healing, soul contracts, and lost worlds back to opening doors to her training as a breathworker and teacher she is today. Again,

continues

her journey has elements unique to her and may or may not be relevant to others. Each of us must find the path that takes us to living our purpose with increased awareness and fulfillment.

"Years ago, I went out to Montana for a five-day silent retreat. I wanted to gain some perspective on what was happening with a long-term relationship. I was madly in love, but I suspected my lover had found someone new. All my fears and betrayal issues came rushing forward, and it was time for some deep therapy. In the silence, in the depths of winter, I came to love myself more. I was ready to face myself, or at least I thought so, and decided to go into couple's counseling with my lover when I returned.

"When I got home, I heard a dog barking. Wait a minute, we don't have a dog, I thought. Lisa opened the door. She was the one I feared was in some kind of relationship with my partner. And she was wearing the emerald-green robe that I had given my lover as a Christmas gift. So, not only was Lisa in my home, her dog was living there! She had moved in over that five-day retreat!

"They made a space for me up in the attic—a futon on the floor with a small chest as a bedside table. There was a lamp, plenty of blankets to keep me warm, even my grandmother's rocking chair was in a corner. The space heater would keep the room from getting frosty. They were trying to make me feel comfortable with an impossible situation.

"I went into shock, crying myself to sleep but hardly able to believe or comprehend what was happening. I could come downstairs to use the bathroom and brush my teeth, they said, but essentially, I would have my own area. I could stay there as long as I wanted and use the facilities, even the kitchen, when they weren't around. Since they both worked, this would give me ample time during the day to have the flat to myself while I went to college.

"About this time, a friend was in breathwork school. When she learned of my situation, she asked if she could work with me, free of charge, for the next six months. She needed the practice. I readily agreed because I needed help!

"In breathwork, after a several deep and profound breaths just to get settled, we came up with an intention. I would work on understanding and

continues

releasing my betrayal issues. That much was obvious. The breath would reveal the healing.

"After a good while into the session of more deep and connected breathing, I started to slip into a superconscious, dreamlike state of mind. She asked me quietly, where was I?

"I told her Lemuria and I repeated it for her. Lemuria. I could tell she was writing it down, because neither of us had heard this word before. She asked me to stay with it and describe what I was experiencing.

"I said, 'There's fire. There has just been a volcano and earthquake I think. People are running for their lives.'

"'Lemuria, Lemuria, I am so sorry,' I cried out as I was watching the scene unfold. And then, more quietly, 'I have to go now … we are gathering.'

"'Who is gathering?' she asked.

"'The Council. I am part of the council, and it is time to leave. We have done all we could. Some people will be lost and will never return, but we must go now.'

"'What else is happening? Stay with it.'

"I told her that we were going up through the tops of our heads. We have learned a technique to breathe and escape from our bodies through the vibration of breath. We are in star space now. We are twelve. There is a circle of twelve of us, but we don't have bodies anymore. We are just circles of light. We are each a little different in our color and intensity, but we are energy balls of radiance, and we are intelligences. We each have our own unique energy signature.

"'Keep feeling it, breathe. What else?'

"'Oh, my God, there is Lisa! I recognize Lisa! She's here, and we have made an agreement. I somehow betrayed her earlier in this lifetime. I took on a lover that she also loved, and I made an agreement that she could do the same for me another time. The same for me.' I knew it was nothing done to me. I see it now. It is and always has been for me.

"'This whole journey, this entire enterprise of existence is for us. Not against. I realized I was not being betrayed by Lisa. I am in the same configuration of celestial beings, the same tribe in fact! I had made this agreement with her, and I recognized her by the energy signature she was

continues

vibrating. We are truly a part of the same circle ... the circle that goes on and on and extends beyond any constriction of the personality."

"I started coming to and making sense of this extraordinary, out-of-body experience. I was at peace, breathing peace, and I have found a new home. I was sheltered now in a brightly lit apartment with a female co-worker. She agreed she could use a roommate for a while. I had nothing to forgive Lisa because I knew we had agreed to this. I had nothing to hold against my former partner either. But what was this place called Lemuria? It still didn't make any sense.

"This was long before the internet, and the term wasn't in the dictionary. But we eventually found reference to it in *The Women's Encyclopedia of Myths and Secrets*. Lemuria was associated with the lost world of Atlantis, said to be a ghost world. We were on fire with recognition! It wasn't just my imagination anymore; it was a real word, even if it was a 'ghost world.' So maybe we are just ghosts! Certainly we are spirits housed in these amazing vehicles ... our bodies. Spirits or energy balls in form.

"Three days later, I was at a friend's house. We were practicing massage and bodywork with a few crystals. It was part of another class I was doing, learning how to give partner massage. It was here I notice a book on her counter with the title of Lemuria right in front. Oh my God! Another lightbulb moment!

"'Where did you get this book?' I asked, 'Can I borrow it? I have to have this book!' I told them of the recent 'rebirth' experience I had.

"I flipped open the pages and turned to maybe the fifth chapter at random ... and what I recall reading was something like this: 'we went up on cords of light, through the tops of our heads, and watched the destruction of the Mother Land. We became balls of energy and gathered with the rest of the Council.'

"I wept in relief, reading these words. Where does this come from? How does it happen? I was twenty-seven years old then, and I needed to read this book. But my host said they couldn't lend it out because it belonged to Harry.

"'Harry?' I asked. 'Not the same Harry that lived with Lisa, by any chance ... before she moved into our place?'

"'Yes. That Harry. You know him. It's his book.'

continues

"It was hard to take this all in. Things were really lining up. Here's this whole book, and the chapter I open up to has a message from my soul. I'm here to work on my betrayal issues. And of all the people in the city that this book could belong to, it happens to be in the same house that my former lover's girlfriend just moved from.

"These synchronistic events are mind-blowing to me and more evidence in this world there is much more at work than can be explained by our everyday existence. This world truly shows up for our discovery. The subconscious mind can be activated to heal ourselves through breathwork. I became more awake and aware because of this process. Here was evidence in my experience that I am truly not alone. And that lifetime after lifetime, we play out roles for one another ... agreements so the soul can grow.

"There was no way I knew this or could know this consciously, and it helped melt all the defenses and places of denial, hurt, and anger that I had. Having this perspective in my mind's eye, with a vision awakened in me through the breath ... turned me unto learning about doing my own breathwork training. I want and still desire to learn and master the workings of the mind. Breathwork is key to this discovery.

"Let me say a bit more of this former partner. We remained friends after this. I see that I was never truly harmed. I wanted to be in contact with the children we lived with. They were growing up so fast. I moved down the street, only a few doors away and got to see them often. It's amazing what forgiveness offers, and opening up to the power of the breath did this for me. There is a deeper mystery at work always supporting us for our own good. Breathe."

Conclusion and Future Developments

In our exploration of breathwork in this book I first presented the science and art of Therapeutic Breathwork as an invaluable adjunct to the practice of counseling and other healing arts. I then talked about its principles and role in the community and traced the roots of the relationship between modern-day counseling and breathwork. I detailed advances in the ways healing trauma is addressed in counseling and breathwork's significant role in this. I covered how developmental body themes present different breathing patterns and the differential approaches Therapeutic Breathwork uses to optimize breathing in each. In this final chapter, I showed you Therapeutic Breathwork's application in life challenges, professional practice, and conscious growth.

In recent years I have attended and presented at a number of conferences that have highlighted the growing areas of research, theory, and application of breathwork from clinical studies to international disaster relief[63] (such as conferences presented by Omega Institute in 2013 and 2014 and Kripalu Center in 2015). The breadth of this emerging field is partially chronicled in *The Complete Breath*.[64] It appears that breath is finally getting its due. Every area of human endeavor in which breath takes a vital role is now becoming a subject of serious study from diagnosis through maintenance to peak performance. What was once a specialized corner of the scientific world dealing with clinical disorders is on its way to becoming a legitimate field unto itself.

I believe this is because of a scientific paradigm shift from subspecialization to integrative approaches. I have called breathwork the "rainbow bridge" that joins realms of the physical, mental, emotional, and spiritual. In many ways we are just bringing breathwork into mainstream awareness. Health maintenance and improvement—physical and mental—now focuses on proper breathing. Yoga, aerobic exercise, jogging, and the great variety of sports all highlight the importance of breath modulation. Most forms of meditation, contemplation, and centering all utilize breath awareness. These are the inroads to contemporary consciousness.

Some of us who have been in the field for years and witnessed the transformative power of breathwork with our clients, students, and communities allow ourselves to dream further to a larger vision of the Spirit of Breath itself as a director of planetary healing and ascension. My codirector of the Global Professional Breathwork Alliance and the founding director of the Breath Immersion: From Science to Samadhi Omega and Kripalu Conferences, Jessica Dibb, uses the term *unified breath field* to describe that which animates all life and links together the awareness of conscious beings into a more creative and compassionate collaboration. She says, "Practicing breathing with conscious awareness and cultivation of the unified breath field ultimately is the hope for humanity out of the path of illusory separation to cocreating and building a world in which all beings can thrive and contribute their gifts to one another." If life on Earth begins and ends with breath, it certainly is a likely candidate for a unifying principle.

All these visions and possibilities start first with breath initiated by loving intention—which is my shorthand definition of breathwork. From this perspective, breathing life into our loving intentions for the world is our common purpose for being on this planet. Consciously breathing together is what will put us back in the driver's seat of our destiny. No one knows what is around every corner, but I firmly believe that having our hands on the wheel and trusting the guidance system of the originating principle of life itself puts us in a better position than unconsciously plunging ahead with one foot on the gas of need and the other on the brake of fear. It has been said that there are no accidents (because we can learn from everything). But if conscious breathing can heighten my self-awareness and presence on the road of life, I'd prefer to learn my lessons by minimizing the crashes my unconsciousness invites.

I invite you as you come to the end of this book to breathe your life into whatever has inspired you in its contents. If there are no accidents in your reading this manuscript, what lessons does your Spirit of Breath draw from it, and what meaning does it have for your life? For my part I am grateful that you have joined me on this journey and look forward to what worlds we will cocreate together.

Breathing with you,
Jim Morningstar

Appendix I

Global Professional Breathwork Alliance's Training Standards and Ethics

The Global Professional Breathwork Alliance (GPBA), established in 2001, is a consortium of professional schools, trainers, and practitioners who support and promote the integration of breathwork in the world as an accessible and vital healing modality that facilitates physical, emotional, intellectual, and spiritual wellness (*http://breathworkalliance.com*). The GPBA's principal mission is to be a standard bearer for profession ethics and training standards in the field of dyadic breathwork.

A. GPBA Principles for Breathworkers

The following are GPBA's principles for breathworkers.

1. Commitment

Unconditional positive regard is one of the most powerful therapeutic healing agents. Breathworkers are committed to an attitude of unconditional love and positive regard for clients, themselves, and other practitioners.

2. Responsibility

a) Breathwork is a method of self-healing and self-empowerment. A breathworker must inform clients of the necessity to be self-motivated and accept personal responsibility for their own transformational process.

b) Breathwork practitioners commit to ongoing personal growth and spiritual development, caring for their bodies, mind, emotions, and spirit.

3. Dedication

Breathworkers are dedicated to the highest good of themselves and others as well as planetary wellness, wholeness, and peace.

4. Inclusion

a) Breathworkers do not discriminate based on race, ethnicity, gender, religion, sexual orientation, age, or appearance.

b) Membership in the Global Professional Breathwork Alliance (GPBA) is meant to be inclusive, inspiring, and supportive in reflecting the highest intention of the collective consciousness of the breathwork community.

5. Excellence

a) Acknowledging ourselves as breathworkers involves receiving the necessary training and continuous involvement in the breathwork community.

b) A professional breathworker is committed to excellence and continuing education and supervision for professional enhancement.

6. Mutuality

A professional breathworker accepts and offers honest constructive feedback with colleagues in settings of mutual agreement (e.g., trainings, conferences, meetings, exchanges, etc.).

7. Integrity

Breathwork involves personal growth and expanded states of consciousness and requires a high level of personal integrity, keeping the welfare of the client as the primary focus.

8. Respect

Breathworkers' values are shared only in the context of respect for the sacredness of the client's unique process and in deference to the client's right to choose his or her own values.

B. Code of Ethics

Breathwork schools, trainers, practitioners, and trainees in the GPBA agree to observe the following code of ethics.

1. Client Suitability

a) Establish a client's ability to utilize and healthfully integrate breathwork, as far as is possible.

b) Not discriminate on the basis of race, ethnicity, gender, religion, sexual orientation, age, or appearance.

2. Contract with Clients

a) Establish clear contracts with clients regarding the number and duration of sessions and financial terms.

b) Establish clear boundaries and discuss the possible employment of touch.

c) Practice my breathwork skills primarily for the benefit of the client, rather than solely for financial gain.

d) Maintain confidentiality of client information and security of records of client session content.

3. Practitioner Competence

a) Practice within my area of professional competence, training, and expertise; make this clear to my prospective clients; and not make claims for my service that cannot be substantiated.

b) Continue to develop personally, practicing the technique that I offer to others while nourishing passion and reverence for my calling, and keeping a healthy balance in my work and self-care.

c) Seek supervision and consultation when appropriate.

4. Practitioner/Client Relationship

a) Establish and maintain healthy, appropriate, and professional boundaries, respecting the rights and dignity of those I serve.

b) Refrain from using my influence to exploit or inappropriately exercise power over my clients.

c) Refrain from using my breathwork practice to promote my personal religious beliefs.

d) Refrain from all forms of sexual behavior or harassment with clients even when client initiates or invites such behavior.

e) Provide clients with information about community networking, educational resources, and holistic lifestyle with their consent and within my scope of knowledge.

f) Refer clients to appropriate resources when they present issues beyond my scope of training.

5. Practitioner Interrelationships

a) Maintain and nurture healthy relationships to other breathworkers.

b) Give constructive feedback to other Alliance practitioners who I believe have failed to follow one or more of the ethical principles. If this does not sufficiently resolve the issue, seek consultation with the most appropriate professional and/or civil authorities within my local region for the protection of breathwork clients involved.

Appendix II

Breathworker Training

Therapeutic Breathwork: Transformations Breathwork Training Program (TBTP)

The purpose of TBTP, founded in 1990, is to train professionals in the art and science of Therapeutic Breathwork (www.transformationsusa.com /breathworker-training.php). It is one of the longest-standing ongoing contemporary breathworker training programs.

The Transformations Breathwork Training Program is a founding member of the Global Professional Breathwork Alliance, which adheres to agreed-upon principles, ethics, and training standards among well-established breathwork training schools around the world.

Courses are approved by the National Board of Certified Counselors (NBCC) and the National Association of Alcoholism and Drug Abuse Counselors (NAADAC) for professional continuing education in the United States.

Courses (on-site and distance learning) can be applied to a Certificate of Therapeutic Breathwork Studies through the School of Integrative Psychology (www.transformationsusa.com/certificate-programs.php) or to academic credit through affiliation with Akamai University (www.akamaiuniversity.us /IntegrativePsychology.html).

JIM MORNINGSTAR, PHD
Director, Transformations Incorporated

jim@transformationsusa.com
www.transformationsusa.com
www.jimmorningstar.com

The following are certified schools that are part of Global Professional Breathwork Alliance (http://breathworkalliance.com/member-directory /certified-schools):

- Avalon Institute of Rebirthing/Ecole Européenne du Souffle Conscient (www.rebirther.co.uk)
- BioDynamic Breath and Trauma Release Institute (www.biodynamicbreath.com)
- Breathwork Trainings International (www.breathworktrainings.com.au)
- Clarity Breathwork (http://claritybreathwork.com/professional-training-program/)
- Ecole Etre (www.ecole-etre.com, www.judeegee.com)
- Eupsychia Institute (www.eupsychia.com/breathwork/)
- Graduate School of Breathing Sciences (www.breathingsciences.bp.edu)
- Holotropic Breathwork (www.holotropic.com/transtrain.shtml)
- Inspiration Consciousness School and Community (www.InspirationCommunity.org)
- Institute for Integrative Breath Therapy (www.breathworkeurope.com)
- International Breathwork Foundation: Schools and Organizations (www.ibfnetwork.com/members/organisations)
- International Center of Conscious Breathing, Studying and Practicing (www.odyhanie.ru)
- Optimal Breathing Mastery (www.breathing.com)
- Power of Breath Institute (www.powerofbreath.com)
- SOURCE Process and Breathwork (www.sourcebreath.com, www.ecstaticbirth.com)
- Transformational Breathwork (http://transformationalbreath.com)
- Transformations Incorporated (www.transformationsusa.com)
- Zentium International Breathwork Mastery (breathworkmastery.com)

Appendix III

Breathwork Research Resources

The following are breathwork research resources:

- Global Professional Breathwork Alliance
  (*http://breathworkalliance.com/resources/breathwork-techniques-research*)
- Holotropic Breathwork
  (*www.grof-holotropic-breathwork.net/page/research-on-holotropic*)
- Lampman, C. and Morningstar, J Compilation of articles on breathing and breathwork
  (*www.transformationsusa.com/Breathwork-Research.pdf*)
- Optimal Breathing Mastery
  (*www.breathing.com/articles/clinical-studies.htm*)

Notes

Introduction

1) Fried, R. 1990. *The Breath Connection*. New York, NY: Insight Books.
2) Minett, G. 2004. *Exhale*. Edinburgh, UK: Floris Books.
3) Lewis, D. 1997. *The Tao of Natural Breathing*. San Francisco, CA: Mountain Wind Publishing.
4) Litchfield, P. 2003. "A Brief Overview of the Chemistry of Respiration and the Breathing Heart Wave." *California Biofeedback* vol. 19, no. 1.
5) HeartMath Institute. 2015. *Science of the Heart: Exploring the Role of the Heart in Human Performance*. https://www.heartmath.org/resources/downloads/science-of-the-heart/
6) Siegel, D. 2012. *The Developing Mind: How Relationships and the Brain Interact to Shape Who We Are*, 2nd ed. New York, NY: Guilford.

Chapter 1

7) Rajski, P. 2002. *International Journal for the Advancement of Counseling* 24 (2).
8) McKeown, P. 2004. *Close Your Mouth: Buteyko Breathing Clinic Self-Help Manual*. County Galway, Ireland: Buteyko Books.
9) Grof, S. 2000. *Psychology of the Future*. Albany, NY: SUNY Press.
10) Taylor, K. 1995. *The Ethics of Caring*. Santa Cruz, CA: Hanford Mead.
11) Morningstar, J. 2001. "Breathwork: Therapy of Choice for Whom?" In *The Spirit of Breathwork*. Cambridge, UK: International Breathwork Foundation.

Chapter 2

12) Morningstar, J. 2014. *Therapeutic Breathwork Introduction and Live Demonstration – Video*. Milwaukee, WI: Transformations Incorporated. http://www.transformationsusa.com/lifelong-learning.php.

Chapter 3

13) Beck, D., and C. Cowen. 1996. *Spiral Dynamics*. Cambridge, MA: Blackwell Publishers.

14) Graves, C., and C. Cowan. 2005. *The Never-Ending Quest: A Treatise on an Emergent Cyclical Conception of Adult Behavioral Systems and Their Development*. Santa Barbara, CA: ECLET Pub.

15) Morningstar, J. 1980, 1998. "Levels of Existence Inventory 'The Way I See It.'" In *Spiritual Psychology*, 3rd ed. Milwaukee, WI: Transformations Incorporated. http://kevinmooresoftware.com /twisiv1/Survey.asp?ID=284435&ST=1'.

16) Shapiro, F. 2001. *Eye Movement Desensitization and Reprocessing: Basic Principles, Protocols, and Procedures*. New York, NY: Guildford Press.

17) Feinstein, D., and D. Eden. 2005. *The Promise of Energy Psychology: Revolutionary Tools for Cramatic Personal Change*. NY: Penguin.

18) Rand, A. 1957. *Atlas Shrugged*. New York, NY: Random House.

19) Freud, S. 1962. *Civilization and Its Discontents*. New York, NY: W.W. Norton.

20) Orne, M. 1962. *Psychological Factors in Maximizing Self-Control under Stress with Special Reference to Hypnosis and Related States*. Ft. Belvoir, VA: Defense Technical Information Center.

21) Jung, C., and Read, H. 1953. *The Collected Works of C. G. Jung*. New York, NY: Pantheon Books.

22) Adler, A. 1927. *Understanding Human Nature*. New York, NY: Greenberg.

23) Rank, O. 1958. *Beyond Psychology*. New York, NY: Dover Publications.

24) Tolman, E. 1966. *Behavior and Psychological Man: Essays in Motivation and Learning*. Berkeley, CA: University of California Press.

25) Rotter, J. 1954. *Social Learning and Clinical Psychology*. New York, NY: Prentice-Hall.

26) Sullivan, H. S. 1953. *The Interpersonal Theory of Psychiatry.* New York, NY: Norton.

27) Kelly, G. 1963. *A Theory of Personality: The Psychology of Personal Constructs.* New York, NY: W. W. Norton.

28) Ellis, A., and D. Ellis. 2011. *Rational Emotive Behavior Therapy.* Washington, DC: American Psychological Association.

29) Lamb, S. D. 2014. *Pathologist of the Mind: Adolf Meyer and the Origins of American Psychiatry.* Baltimore, MD: Johns Hopkins University Press.

30) Horney, K. 1967. *Feminine Psychology: Papers.* New York, NY: W. W. Norton.

31) Erikson, E. 1964. *Childhood and Society,* 2nd ed. New York, NY: Norton.

32) Fromm, E. 1973. *The Anatomy of Human Destructiveness.* New York, NY: Henry Holt.

33) Satir, V. 1967. *Conjoint Family Therapy: A Guide to Theory and Technique,* rev. ed. Palo Alto, CA: Science and Behavior Books.

34) Jackson, D. 1964. *Myths of Madness: New Facts for Old Fallacies.* New York, NY: Macmillan.

35) Bateson, G. 1979. *Mind and Nature: A Necessary Unity.* New York, NY: Dutton.

36) Perls, F. 1969. *In and Out the Garbage Pail.* Lafayette, CA: Real People Press.

37) Shaffer, J., and M. Galinsky. 1974. *Models of Group Therapy and Sensitivity Training.* Englewood Cliffs, NJ: Prentice-Hall.

38) Lowen, A. 1975. *Bioenergetics.* New York, NY: Coward, McCann & Geoghegan.

39) Rolf, I., and R. Feitis. 1978. *Ida Rolf Talks about Rolfing and Physical Reality.* New York, NY: Harper & Row.

40) Rolf, I. 1977. *Rolfing: The Integration of Human Structures* Santa Monica, CA: Dennis-Landman.

41) Grof, S., and C. Grof. 2010. *Holotropic Breathwork: A New Approach to Self-Exploration and Therapy.* Albany, NY: State University of New York Press.

42) Rogers, C. 1951. *Client-Centered Therapy: Its Current Practice, Implications, and Theory.* Boston, MA: Houghton Mifflin.

43) Maslow, A. 1971. *The Farther Reaches of Human Nature.* New York, NY: Viking Press.

44) Wilber, K. 2000. *Integral Psychology: Consciousness, Spirit, Psychology, Therapy.* Boston, MA: Shambhala.

45) Grof, S. 2000. *Psychology of the Future Lessons from Modern Consciousness Research.* Albany, NY: State University of New York Press.

Chapter 4

46) Levine, P. 2008. *Healing Trauma: A Pioneering Program for Restoring the Wisdom of Your Body.* Boulder, CO: Sounds True.

47) Siegel, D. 2010. *Mindsight: The New Science of Personal Transformation.* New York, NY: Bantam.

48) van der Kolk, B. 2014. *The Body Keeps the Score.* New York, NY: Penguin.

49) Linehan, M. 2014. *DBT Skills Training Manual.* New York, NY: Guilford.

50) Feinstein, D., and D. Eden. 2005. *The Promise of Energy Psychology.* New York, NY: Penguin.

51) Naparstek, B. 2004. *Invisible Heroes: Survivors of Trauma and How They Heal.* New York, NY: Bantam.

52) Andrade, C., and R. Radhakrishnan. 2009. "Prayer and Healing: A Medical and Scientific Perspective on Randomized Controlled Trials." *Indian Journal of Psychiatry* 51(4): 247–253.

Chapter 5

Thanks to Joanna Farina, MA, for her input in compiling the research for this chapter.

53) Siegel, D. J. 2001. "Toward an Interpersonal Neurobiology of the Developing Mind: Attachment Relationships, 'Mindsight,' and Neural Integration." *Infant Mental Health Journal* 22(1–2): 67–94.

54) Schore, A. N. 2001. "The Effects of Early Relational Trauma on Right Brain Development, Affect Regulation, and Infant Mental Health." *Infant Mental Health Journal* 22(1–2): 201–269.

55) Stern, D. N. 1985. *The Interpersonal World of the Infant.* New York, NY: Basic Books.

56) Porges, S. W. 2001. "The Polyvagal Theory: Phylogenic Substrates of a Social Nervous System." *International Journal of Psychophysiology* 42:123–146.

57) Glazer, R., and H. Friedman. 2010. "Bioenergetic Therapy." *The Corsini Encyclopedia of Psychology* vol. 2010: 234–235, 1800–1802.

58) Morningstar, J. 1980/1998. *Spiritual Psychology*, 3rd ed. Milwaukee: Transformations Incorporated.

59) Joseph, R. 1999. "Environmental Influences on Neural Plasticity, the Limbic System, Emotional Development and Attachment: A Review." *Child Psychiatry and Human Development* 29(3).

60) Bentzen, M. 2006. "Shapes of Experience: Neuroscience, Developmental Psychology and Somatic Character Formation." In *Handbook of Bodypsychotherapy*. Schattauer.

61) Glazer, R., and H. Friedman. 2009. "The Construct Validity of the Bioenergetics-Analytic Character Typology: A Multi-Method Investigation of a Humanistic Approach to Personality." *The Humanistic Psychologist* 37: 24–48.

62) Porges, S. W. 2003. Social Engagement and Attachment: A Phylogenic Perspective. *Annals New York Academy of Science* 1008:31–47.

Chapter 6

63) Gerbarg, P., and R. Brown. 2012. *Breath Body Mind Training Efficacy in Mass Disasters, Trauma, and Community Resilience in the Complete Breath*. Milwaukee, WI: Transformations Incorporated.

64) Morningstar, J. 2012. *The Complete Breath*. Milwaukee, WI: Transformations Incorporated.

Index

About the Author

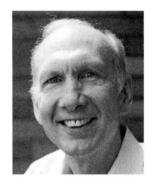

Jim Morningstar, PhD, is the originator of Therapeutic Breathwork™, director of one of the longest-standing breathwork training centers in the world, and codirector and founder of the Global Professional Breathwork Alliance, which sets ethical and training standards for the field of dyadic breathwork.

As director of Transformations Incorporated, Morningstar has held licensure as a clinical psychologist since 1973, receiving distinguished honors as an ABPP practitioner five years later. He has been a member of the American Psychological Association since 1975 and was an assistant clinical professor in the Department of Psychiatry and Mental Health Sciences at the Medical College of Wisconsin from 1977 to 1989. He is a clinical supervisor and seminar leader and has pioneered in the integration of psychotherapy with such mind-body techniques as breathwork and biospiritual energetics. He founded the School of Integrative Psychology in 1980 and the Transformations Breathworker Training Program in 1990 and has authored four books in the field of psychology and breathwork: *Family Awakening* (1984), *Spiritual Psychology* (rev. 1998), *Breathing in Light and Love* (1994, revised ebook 2015), and *The Complete Breath: A Professional Guide to Health and Wellbeing* (2012).

Morningstar's lifelong quest has been to discover and teach the highest-quality tools for human transformation. He has done this as a clinical psychologist, spiritual student/teacher, trainer and lecturer, author, and personal growth and business coach for almost half a century.

About North Atlantic Books

North Atlantic Books (NAB) is an independent, nonprofit publisher committed to a bold exploration of the relationships between mind, body, spirit, and nature. Founded in 1974, NAB aims to nurture a holistic view of the arts, sciences, humanities, and healing. To make a donation or to learn more about our books, authors, events, and newsletter, please visit www.northatlanticbooks.com.

For more information on books, authors, events, and to sign up for our newsletter, please visit www.northatlanticbooks.com.

North Atlantic Books is the publishing arm of the Society for the Study of Native Arts and Sciences, a 501(c)(3) nonprofit educational organization that promotes cross-cultural perspectives linking scientific, social, and artistic fields. To learn how you can support us, please visit our website.